The **Louise Parker** Method

LE̶ ̶FE

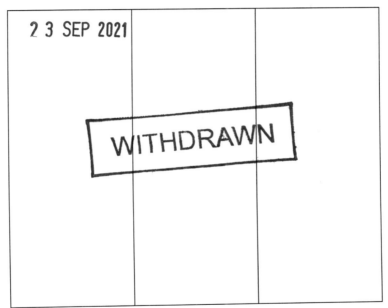

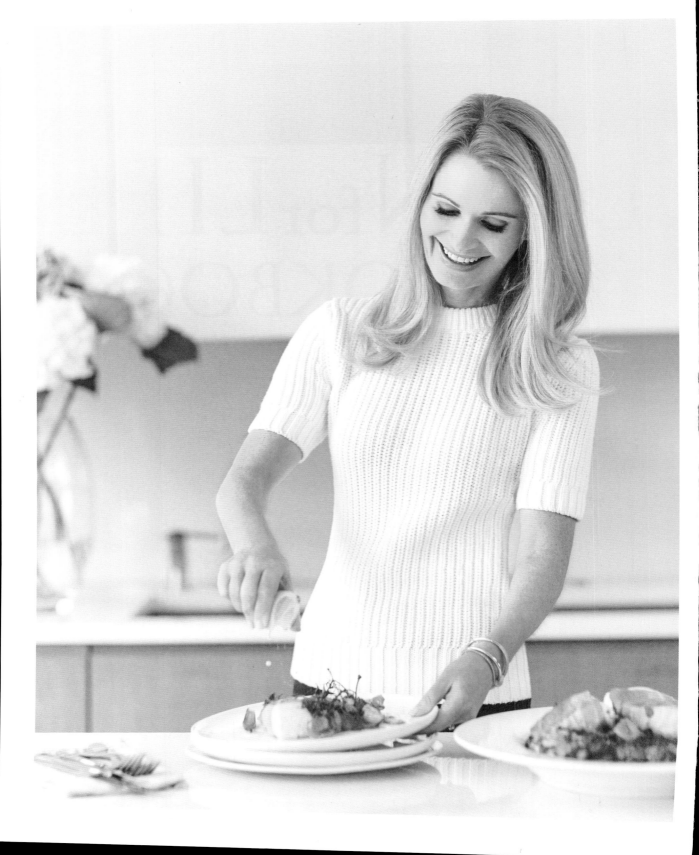

The **Louise Parker** Method

LEAN for LIFE
The COOKBOOK

MITCHELL BEAZLEY

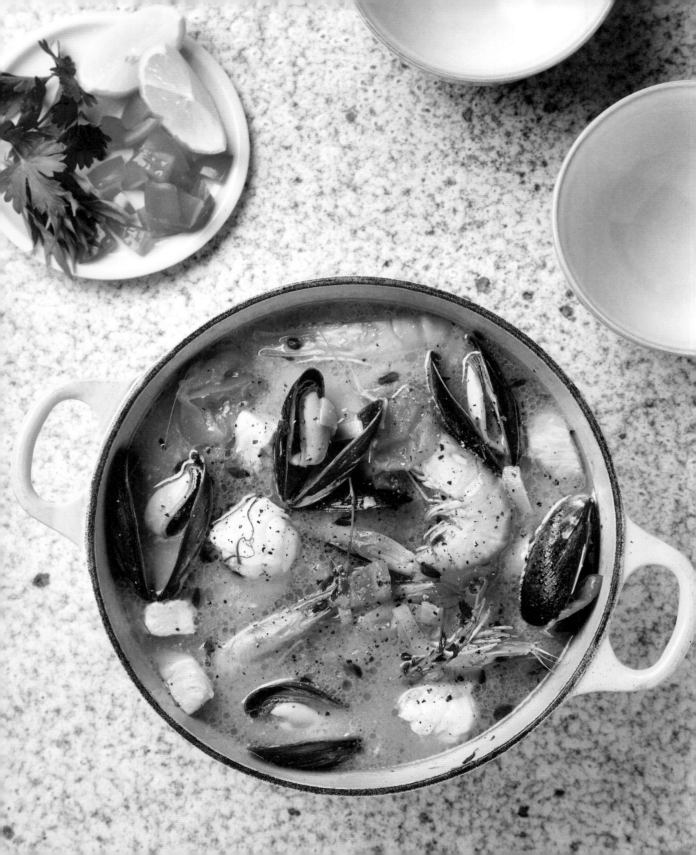

CONTENTS

INTRODUCTION

I loathe dieting. I'm actually on a mission to end it. By the time my three daughters are grown up, I'd like them to think it as absurd as smoking was on planes, not so very long ago. I hope that, when I confess I did both, they'll be horrified.

Dieting is deprivation, tediously boring and doesn't even work. I spent a decade of my life in a body trapped in fad diets, false promises and with a backside I thank God was behind me. I allowed what I ate, what I didn't eat and what I weighed to define my mood each day. That's a lot of wasted hours that I'll never get back. The upside is, I've got a PhD in hindsight that I now put to good use.

For some, eating in balance is intuitive. But for millions of us, we unlearn good habits by the time we first 'diet', or never learn them in the first place. The Louise Parker Method is the lifestyle that gets you the body you want and sustains you there, in optimum health and brimming with vitality. The side-effect of this lifestyle is that your body will transform into one that is exceptionally lean, sculpted, strong and graceful. And because you've changed the habits of your lifestyle, the results stick. It will become part of you, not something that crashes to a grinding halt.

In my first book, *The Louise Parker Method: Lean For Life*, I introduced you to the four pillars of our Method and the programme to help you Transform. They are: Think Successfully; Live Well; Eat Beautifully; and Work Out Intelligently. In this book, I share many more recipes that I hope will become part of your family repertoire and give you the ideas and inspiration to help you 'Eat Beautifully'... and utterly enjoy your Lean for Life lifestyle.

For the most part, I want fit, fast food and my first book offered my speedier, most practical meals. Here I'm going to share with you a blend of many more quickies, as well as some requiring just a bit more time and and effort, so that you can have a wider repertoire.

Now, I'm the first to admit I am no chef. I do, however, love good food. I love how it turns a house into a home, a gathering into a party, and socially glues friends and family together. I think it should always be celebrated, whether it's a quick Monday morning breakfast or a long, lazy Sunday brunch with friends. We rush through life, and a little meal or snack just punctuates our days with a little pleasure, and forces us to stop.

I learned to cook in my mother's kitchen. Her passion and skill far outweigh my own. Growing up on a farm in South Africa, I'd help milk the cows and watch her churn her own butter, make her own cheese, and throw the most sensational dinner parties. I learned all the basics of cooking, hanging off her homemade Biba-inspired dresses in a house my father built in Ladysmith, Natal. Mealtimes were set in stone – with a beautifully laid table whatever the occasion – and so from an early age it was instilled in me that meals were about celebration, conversation, family and friends, and always, always laughter. School years in the Middle East and, later, travel in my twenties introduced me to flavours and street foods I still salivate over, and have certainly influenced how I cook and what my family eat today.

The Louise Parker Method is 20 years in the making. During the first 10, I devised my first programme, The Intensive, and taught it personally to hundreds of clients. It grew by word of mouth and, for the last decade, my team and I have delivered thousands of programmes worldwide. It's truly tried and tested – we've seen success even in the most challenging of life situations – and I know that if you really want it, it will work for you.

I hope that you love Eating Beautifully, find the same liberation from dieting as I have, and – best of all – discover the blueprint for permanent success.

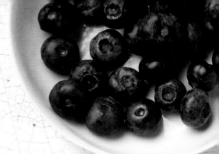

TESTIMONIALS FOR LOUISE'S FIRST BOOK

I know that this Method works because this is the way that I live and this is the way that thousands of people have found that they can lose fat, have a lean body and keep it that way for good.

One of the most satisfying things is hearing from those who are successfully living the Louise Parker Method.

Here are just a few testimonials. Check out our website and Instagram for more.

Anna, 45

'Having tried every diet out there, I wanted it all: a method that was simple to follow, effective and sustainable, and delicious food that kept me trim and healthy. Lean for Life is that and SO much more!
'Losing the weight was great but the liberation from dieting and increased energy levels are just a few of the other long-lasting benefits. I've loved the journey and I love my new "normal". 'Thank you so much @louiseparkermethod for creating such an inspirational book. Quite simply life changing!'

Wendy, 54

'The choices of delicious meals are simply stunning. Another plus is how quick the recipes are to make and all add a maximum flavour-punch to each meal. I have no hesitation about serving any dish for guests – they have no idea they're "on programme" when they come to visit.'

Tricia, 65

'Over the last 30 years I had been on every diet, was unhealthy and unfit. Your book was such an easy read and it just made complete sense. I have done two of the six weeks, have lost 25lbs and not found it difficult. Thank you Louise!'

Kate, 29

'If I can lose 20lbs whilst living and eating out in NYC then anyone can. I'm now in the best shape of my life. Thank you to Louise Parker for the freedom from trend dieting. Don't pick and mix, if you follow the four pillars and assume success, it can't not work!'

Louise, 41

'After nine and a half weeks in the Transform phase, I had lost 24lbs and 21½ inches from various parts of my body. I no longer feel bloated, my cellulite has disappeared and my skin is glowing. I love my new figure!
'The physical changes are amazing but the Method has changed me mentally. I feel so positive, healthy and, importantly, happy. So a huge thank you @louiseparkermethod and the online tribe who have been an invaluable support throughout my journey.'

Becky, 41

'All I can say is WOW! Words cannot express how much you have changed my life, I was so happy this morning when I weighed myself and saw how much I had lost, that I cried!'

Our Method isn't a 'diet'. It's a lifestyle that will become a part of you

THE LOUISE PARKER METHOD

If you read my first book, you'll be familiar with the basics. The Louise Parker Method is a lifestyle, a habit, an attitude and not a diet. It's a style of living that perfectly blends Eating Beautifully, Working Out Intelligently, Thinking Successfully and Living Well. It's a real-life solution to permanent weight loss and optimum health, while allowing all the pleasures of life – in moderation – to keep you sane and happy.

There are two phases.

We start with the Transform Phase, lasting 42 days. Depending on how far you have to travel, you complete one round, two rounds, or as many as you need until you reach your ultimate goal. At Louise Parker we run programmes with a minimum of 42 days. These 42 days are crucial. They give your mind the time it needs to really adapt to your new habits, and – of course – to give you the result you want.

Then we ease into the the Lifestyle Phase. All the new habits you learn become part of you and how you live, making it the most effortless lifestyle change possible. You learn balance, and by balance I mean just being able to have a burger and enjoy it for what it is. No celebration, cake or cocktail is off limits. As long as it's 'worth it' to you, enjoy it in perfect balance.

It's the combination of all the four pillars that give our Method the power to transform you, swiftly and simply but – most importantly – it really is sustainable. The Lifestyle Phase is a zone where you'll feel comfortable, happy, celebrate food and life and simply be the very best version of yourself, for ever.

IN THE TRANSFORM PHASE, YOU'LL SIMPLY:

THINK SUCCESSFULLY

★ Adopt a positive mental attitude

★ Assume nothing but success

★ Visualize your goal. It needs to be so clear you can literally feel it

★ Keep positive, inspiring company

1

LIVE WELL

★ Declutter your surroundings

★ Digital detox after 9pm every night

★ Sleep 7–8 hours a night

★ Take a 'brain-nap' for 20 minutes a day

★ Make time for simple pleasures every single day

2

EAT BEAUTIFULLY

★ Eat 3 meals and 2 snacks per day

★ Balance each meal with all the necessary macronutrients – protein, fat and low-GI carbs

★ Stay well hydrated

★ Prepare your meals beautifully

3

WORK OUT INTELLIGENTLY

★ Weave activity into your everyday, with an absolute minimum of 10,000 steps per day. Aim as high as you can.

★ Complete a minimum of 15 minutes of my Louise Parker Method workouts (see *Lean for Life*)

4

THE 4 PILLARS

For the best result, you need balance. Think of the four pillars as legs of a chair. Sit on all four and you're safe. Rely on three and chances are you'll stay up, it's just going to wobble. Two legs and you're going to topple over quickly. One, and you're going to fall on your arse. You get the idea.

1 THINK SUCCESSFULLY

You're going to need to take a huge leap of faith and assume nothing but success. Ditch any 'stinking thinking' (the negative thoughts that can sabotage your success from the inside) and leave any past failures behind you. We're moving on, and not looking back. Visualize success clearly in the 'movies of your mind', so you can literally feel it. Be bold in terms of what you aim for, and aim higher than you think possible. And, most of all, 'Think in Ink', making sure you commit your goals to paper. Make yourself an absolute priority – it's not selfish, it's essential – as no one else is going to do it for you. If you have to, just fake it until you make it.

2 LIVE WELL

You are in control of your lifestyle and so, if it's not working for you, change it. Declutter your surroundings and tackle all those little grey clouds hanging over your head. Work out how to get at least seven hours of sleep a night and actually put a plan in place to achieve that. You'll find a 'Digital Detox' after 9pm helps massively. Have a bath, read a proper book and don't waste time doing things that don't help you reach your goal. Make time for simple pleasures every day and keep uplifting, positive and inspiring company. Take some time out every day – even if just 20 minutes to 'brain nap' – and allow yourself to totally switch off. These simple tweaks create a sense of calm, manage your hormones, optimize weight loss and – most of all – create a new lifestyle that you love so much, you won't want to ever go back.

3 EAT BEAUTIFULLY

Eating Beautifully is the nutrition pillar, and is probably the reason why you've bought this book. It means eating fresh, real food that is beautifully balanced for optimum fat loss, metabolic preservation and total health. We've done the sciencey bit for you in the recipes here, including low-GI carbs, good amounts of metabolism-boosting protein and just the right amount of fat. All you need to do is just follow the principles. In this book, we help you learn the difference between 'eating clean' and 'eating lean' (see page 14). As well as 140 new recipes, we focus on helping you to create your own beautiful style of eating. Buy the best ingredients you can afford, present your food as beautifully as you can and eat each meal with a little bit of celebration.

4 WORK OUT INTELLIGENTLY

Quite simply, you are going to move more and become an active person. We start with just walking, aiming towards 10,000 steps a day. Ease into it. Some days will be better than others, but I call these steps 'paying your daily rent' to your body and it is essential in gaining and maintaining a sculpted, lean figure.

In my first book *Lean for Life* you'll find examples of my cardio-sculpting workouts, which you can do at home without any equipment at all. They focus on sculpting a beautifully balanced, lean physique, while keeping your heart rate up. With high repetitions, your 'fat-burning tap' turns on while we tone you inch by inch. The idea is to engage your whole body in every single workout and ensure that each one boosts your metabolism for a minimum of 24 hours.

THE DANCE

I introduced this concept in my book *Lean for Life* and it's worth repeating here, as I really think it helped to make our method 'click' for so many readers and followers of my first book.

Think of our Method as a sort of dance: when you learn the steps (the four pillars of success, see page 9) and practise them, *they will become part of who you are*, and not 'something you are doing'.

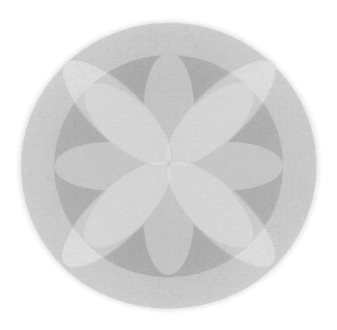

So, imagine an inner circle. This represents the core of our Method and I'd like you to spend as much of your time in this 'inner circle' as possible while you're in the Transform Phase. This isn't because I'm a fitness nerd, but because I want you to take the easy, most direct route to your goal.

Now imagine an outer circle. Once you've reached your goal and switched to the Lifestyle Phase, you're probably going to spend about 20% of your time there, depending on how active you are. You step out when it's worth it, step back, step out, step home… but you always come home again, because this is where you live now. You'll learn what your 'worth its' are and let go of words like 'sins', 'treats' and 'cheats'. And, if you have a blip, recognize it as just that. Don't use a blip as an excuse to give up on something that can potentially change your life, it's just a step in the dance. Simply step back into the inner circle. Essentially, it's about learning not to throw the towel in every time you feel you've been less than perfect. Perfection does not exist and I want you to have a life. We all ebb and flow. We're just going to try and ebb full-on for as long as we can, until you get the habit.

Don't use a blip as an excuse to give up. Simply step back into the inner circle

THE SECRET TO PERMANENT FAT LOSS

Nothing makes me wince more than the term 'New Year, New you'. I know the shelves are awash with 'diet books' in January, but I really think the concept of changing your life is something you can do at any time of year. I don't want to perpetuate the 'diet' movement; I'm really trying to go against the grain of that.

'Now' is always a good time to start, if you are ready. If you're not just yet, digest it a bit, and start when you are. The gyms are packed with good intentions in January and eerily quiet in February. There's a reason for that. You're going to be bombarded with promises every New Year… all I can say, is: please keep your wits about you and know when you're being sold a fad.

Whatever programme you embark on (and I really hope it's ours), ask yourself:

* **Will I still be doing 80% of the principle in five years' time?**

* **Would I allow my teenage daughter to do it?**

If you can answer YES to both these questions, I think you're good to go.

If it's faddy and has a too-good-to-be-true headline, walk on by.

The secret to permanent weight loss is this… *there is no secret.* There's not a cleanse, a detox, a 'superfood' on the planet that will give you lasting results. But if you change your lifestyle and really live the Louise Parker Method, you'll be astonished with both the result and the ease of maintaining it.

We know the fad diets don't work and that there must be a simpler way, but when we're feeling desperate, it's amazing the nonsense we allow ourselves to believe. We all know we need to eat better, sleep more and move more, so why can't we just do it? We want the result now and the promise of a miracle in a week tempts the brightest of us, especially when we're at an all-time low.

With our Method, you *will* get a swift transformation. But I primarily want a forever result for you. Everyone has an initial surge of motivation and willpower, but you can't rely on willpower forever, which is why your new habits are essential.

So how do you keep going after that initial boost? We have to focus on changing your habits. You have to love these habits and, eventually, you'll wear your new lifestyle loosely. If it feels like a pair of control pants, you're going to rip it off,… and we're back to square one.

We need the momentum, the daily practice, until the habits actually become you and you don't have to rely on willpower alone. Motivation is temporary, it always ebbs and flows, while habits last a lifetime. So let's start once and just not stop until you reach your goal. I say this because I know that the easy route is the direct route.

Overleaf is how I've kept the momentum going and helped myself and thousands of others to Transform, both physically and mentally.

Start once

By starting once and never giving up, you take the direct route. You'll hiccup, of course. But that's human: you're not a machine and perfection does not exist. Think of our Method like breathing. When you have days that test you, keep taking shallow breaths – the tiniest effort will be enough to sustain you – until you have a day when you can breathe deeply again.

Know what you want, in technicolour

'I want to lose weight' is not enough. Think in ink and *write* it down: know exactly what you want. It has to be so clear that, when you close your eyes, you can visualize it and actually feel it. Play it over and over in your mind and, when you reach your goal, it should feel like déjà vu. If you can't articulate it and define it with absolute clarity, it's a wish and not a goal.

Before you start your Transform Phase, take time to define your goals and take photos of yourself. This really is the best way for you to see the amazing results you will achieve (it will also allow you to join the exclusive #clownpants club with your results).

Commit to yourself and others

Making yourself accountable to others is a great way to supercharge your initial motivation and staying power. If you don't have cheerleaders within your friends or family, you'll be amazed by the support you will find on social media. I've been stunned by the community on social media, the support is staggering.

Consistency wins the race

Keep practising the steps and, hand on heart, I promise that you will learn our Method and it'll just become part of what you do and how you live. It's just a dance and you need to learn the steps. Know that consistency beats severity every time. Once you're at goal, we teach you the Lifestyle Phase, which is just another step in the dance. Living in true balance really can be taught. Ultimately, the dance is what is going to keep you in your skinny jeans, while still enjoying a damn good life and not becoming a total health and fitness bore.

Re-start your day at any point

Perfection is an illusion. Aim high for sure, but if you step out of the inner circle, the sky will not collapse in on you. You can step back in at any point. Don't write off a whole week because you ate a croissant. Just step back in. The whole point is that we're letting go of a 'diet mentality' and focusing on being consistent. It truly works.

Strive, but know when to go easy on yourself

Treat yourself as you would your child or your friend: mother yourself when you feel you need it. It's not a race. Don't abuse yourself for being imperfect, that's 'stinking thinking' that'll just fuel self-sabotage and talk you into quitting. Erase 'cheat' and 'sins' from your vocabulary. An extra piece of toast is an extra piece of toast. A sin is sleeping with your best friend's husband. Keep perspective.

Celebrate your success

Focus on what you have achieved and not on what you have not. Along the way, treat yourself, but remember that food is never a 'treat'. Break the habit where you celebrate your 'clown pants' with food. Food is not the carrot, nor the stick. It's important you break this link to get out of that 'diet' mentality. Buy yourself flowers, bath salts you can just about afford, a new book, a day off… anything that is going to lift you up. Recognizing how far you've come – broken bad habits, rebuilt lasting healthy ones and overcome hurdles you've faced – is a really important part of your change.

Think in ink. Write it down

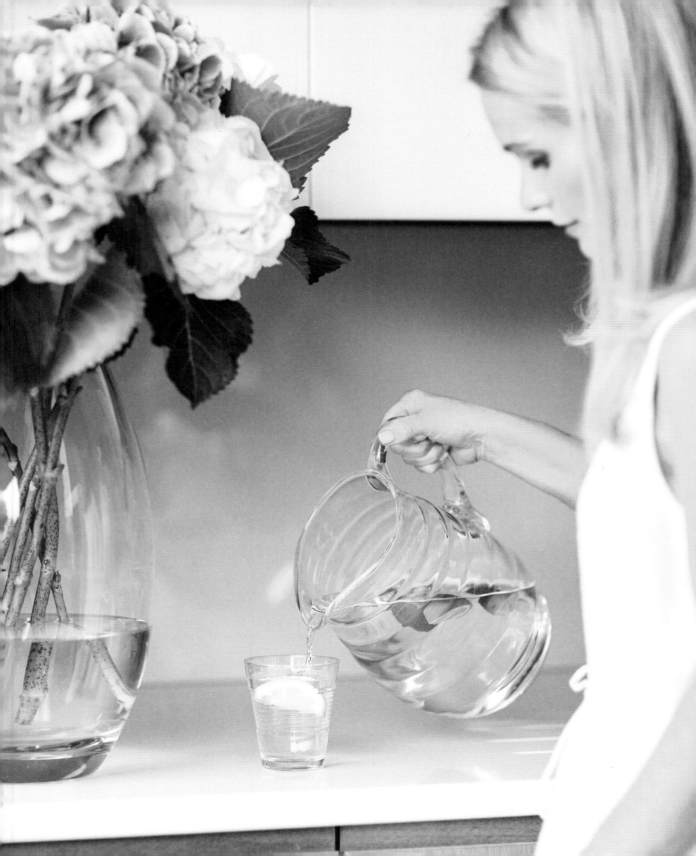

THE DIRT ON 'CLEAN EATING'

Really take this in and you're going to save yourself a mighty amount of time, money and effort… and avoid the 'organically overweight' trap. Remember that weight loss is big business and, everywhere you look, there's a packet of 'everything-free' something – likely organic and hand-picked by vegan virgins – to lure you in. (Some of my best friends are vegan virgins, and organic is great, but you get my point.) You've got to have your wits about you and know when you're being sold something that you're honestly better off without, if your goal is sustainable fat loss.

Remember that every article you read will need an 'angle', and this perpetuates fads. I was once asked to add a raw red onion to my dietary advice in order for an article to hit the press. I didn't, and luckily 'The Red Onion Diet' was never published.

The girl with the super bod on Instagram might be being paid to pour a 'magic drink' down her tanned throat; she may even be air-brushed to hell and back. The fads are oh, so tempting, I know, I've been there. I've done them all. That's why I'm here now: to tell you the truth.

It's not easy to pick out the facts from the hype when you're reading about a quick-fix 'cure', but we're going to get you thinking with your head and not your (temporary) muffin top. Here are the lessons I have learned along the way that I hope will prevent you being 'organically overweight', and sift the fads from the facts.

Not-so-superfood

No food or drink is a 'superfood'. What is 'super' is a balance of all highly nutritious foods; they all bring something to the table. Of course, there are foods that contain an abundance of phytonutrients in comparison to others, and I've included many of these that are easily available in my recipes. Always look at the balance and variety of your whole diet, and not just the amount of one 'good' ingredient: however nutritious something is, there's only so much that one food can do for you. Nothing will transform you into a beacon of health unless you look at the overall balance of what you eat and drink, how you move and how you live.

Calories and portions matter

Your muscle mass determines your metabolism. This, and how much you move, determines how many calories you need. If you're trying to lose body fat then you need a caloric deficit. If you're eating 'healthy halo' foods in abundance – no matter how nutritious – your backside isn't going to thank you for it, however 'natural', 'raw' or 'super' they are. You really can have too much of a good thing. My recipes focus on portions, as calories are way too tedious to count.

Buy the best you can

I am passionate that we should all buy the best produce we can afford, very simply because it tastes better. The quality of what I feed my family matters to me, but that doesn't mean everything I buy is organic. Just because something is organic doesn't mean it's going to be especially nutritious, or help you to get in shape; after all, an organic cake is still a cake. The one area where I do think organic makes a difference is meat. It is an investment, but I think avoiding the hormones and antibiotics in non-organic meat is a plus if you're after fat loss. But, remember, it's only worth it if the rest of your diet is on plan. Eating organic chicken won't help you if you're chasing it up with organic energy balls at 200 calories a pop.

'Healthy food' in disguise

While organic actually means something specific, make sure you kick the tyres on anything labeled 'raw', 'whole' or 'natural'. This might seem contradictory, given that our Method is based on whole foods, but all those buzz words are a marketeer's paradise, as they can be used on almost anything. There are some great products out there, but the trick is to read the label and see what's actually inside the packets. For example, watch out for fructose: it's natural sugar from fruit, but it's still sugar. The best advice is to check how far down the ingredients list any sugars are: the lower down the list, the better.

Swot up

Sadly, there's no easy way round it; doing a little extra research into the foods you eat really does pay off. There is so much misconception out there. Here are some of the most common confusions:

Acai – great for antioxidants and helping to neutralize free radicals (which are produced from fat loss, so antioxidants do support continued fat loss)... but hey, so do blueberries, cranberries, raspberries and strawberries. Often, acai is mixed with other ingredients, including sugars, which supercharge the flavour while also, sadly, adding to your waistline.

Agave – while naturally occurring, the sugars in this super-sweet plant sap are mainly fructose, which is metabolized in the liver and converted into fat stores. It is low-GI, hence its 'wholesome, healthy' reputation, but it's not going to make your bottom smaller. Sugar is sugar, no matter how natural the source, and we want to avoid it most of the time. When you do eat sugar, make sure it's in a crème brûlée or a glass of wine, or something else that's truly worth it for you.

Chia – sadly not magic. It is a seed and you need to eat the same limited amount as you would of other seeds due to the fat content. So eating a huge bowl of it is going to have a high calorific content. Get the portion size right and it is a good protein alternative for vegan and vegetarian diets.

Coconut oil – natural, trendy, fine in moderation... but still not magic. It's less good for both your total cholesterol and the bad type than unsaturated plant-based oils. While it's unbelievably tasty, olive oil is a better bet for weight loss and optimum health.

Dairy – obviously to be avoided if you have a medically identified intolerance to lactose, but not, in my opinion, unhealthy. Calcium and protein both aid fat loss and so it's a fabulous ingredient. Of course, if you don't want to consume it for ethical reasons, that's a different story, and I respect that. But again, kick the tyres of any dairy alternatives; even without added sugar, some contain more sugar and less protein than dairy, so just read the labels and know how much sugar and protein your dairy alternative has.

Gluten-free – essential to avoid if you have coeliac disease, and a smart move if you're gluten-intolerant, but otherwise there's no hard science to support ditching gluten. There's also no proven link to improved weight loss, or health generally, if you go gluten-free, just keep it high-fibre.

Quinoa – Don't confuse 'a source of good protein' with 'high in protein'. Quinoa has a complete amino acid profile, which is essential for a healthy diet, but it's not strictly a high-protein food. It contains good-quality protein, hence the confusion, but, nutritionally, it's not dramatically different to brown rice. So sadly it's not a diet superfood, but it's a good food, especially for vegetarians, that's why it's in my Extra Energy Sides section.

No food or drink is a 'superfood'. What is 'super' is a balance of all highly nutritious foods

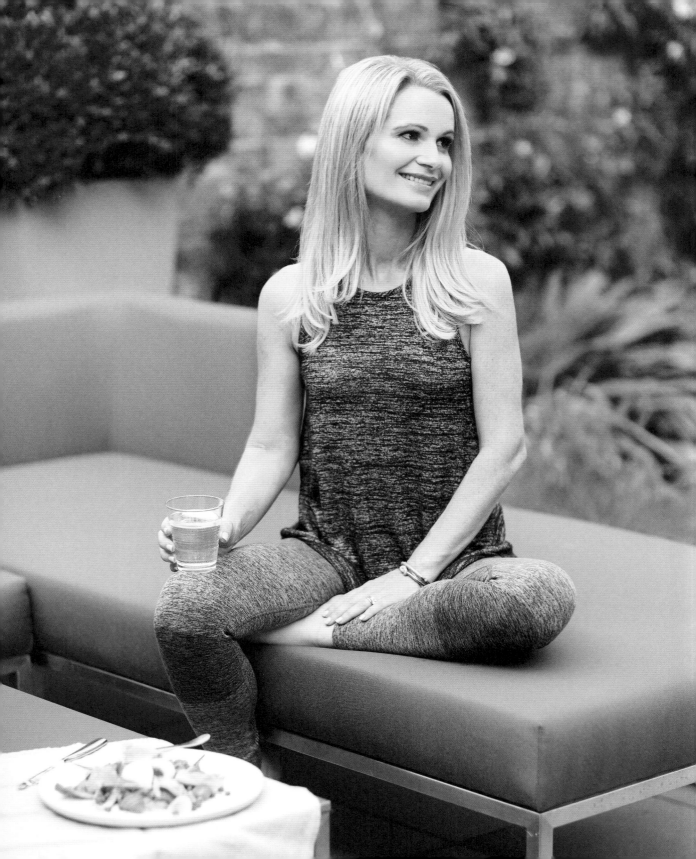

FIND THE TIME TO MOVE

I know how hard it is to find the time to move, train and leap over all the excuses. We are all busy but spending just 15 minutes a day doing less pottering (I'm the number one culprit) allows you time to dedicate to your body. You can honestly make a serious difference in that time. You're going to hate me for this: we all have the time. We just choose to pretend we don't. Find it. It will dramatically change your body *if* you put it to good use. And our Method is about optimizing your result in the minimum time possible.

You can't out-train a bad diet and fat loss is hugely about what you eat. However if you want a sculpted, strong, healthy body, you've simply got to use it. I'm time-poor and so my training needs to slot neatly into my lifestyle instead of taking over and I need the biggest return on my time investment.

10,000 – The magic number

The distance you walk every day is often overlooked in favour of arduous workouts, but it shouldn't be. You need to think of it as something that you will weave into your average day, as it's the basis for so many positive health factors. Ideally, it should just be *'something you do'* and part of your lifestyle rather than a specific activity. It may take a deliberate effort initially but you'll feel a million times better once you have it in place. Track your steps for a fortnight and identify what you need to do to get your movement up. Simple tricks make a big difference; for example I never take a phone call sitting down.

Just pay your daily rent

Aim to do a little exercise every day to build the habit into your life. If you don't stop the exercise habit, then you won't stop. On some days you will put in a higher effort, while on others you may just manage a few squats as the bath is running, but just keep paying your daily rent. You'll find that, over the week, you'll have a good balance. Arduous, grueling workouts are not necessary for a great body. Consistency, however, is. Think about what you're more likely to enjoy and keep it up. Keep changing your repertoire. I change my routine up a bit at the start of every school term and holiday, so six times a year I shock my body and engage my brain so I don't get stuck in a rut.

Focus on the afterburn

If you're time-poor, the most efficient route for you is cardio-sculpting routines, using light weights or bodyweight and high repetitions. You'll tone in a beautifully balanced way and get your heart rate up, so you're combining cardio with conditioning work. It's the best time saver ever and it'll get your afterburn going – this is the rate at which your body burns fat after a session. Don't just focus on what you burn in calories during the session. It's more important we sculpt and strengthen you and get that metabolism up for the 24 hours after each session. Forget counting calories you've stacked up on a treadmill.

Do what you love

If you're trying to boost the amount of exercise you do, especially if it's from a low starting base, do more of what you enjoy. If you play tennis once a week, try to increase it to two. If it's a dance class, try to add in another session. If you enjoy it, you're far more likely to stick at it. I'd love you to do my workouts, but don't feel you have to drop the activities that you are in the habit of doing and love. Do what feels good. But make sure you are strengthening and not just doing cardio: I want you active forever, so you need to find the joy in it. And remember that, even if you focus on activities you enjoy, some days it will feel just like taking your medicine, and that's OK too. Just take it; don't overthink it and swallow it quickly.

Accept the challenge

If exercise is always going to be a little like medicine for you – to be endured rather than enjoyed – then try buddying up with a friend, or signing up for a challenge. It may feel daunting or embarrassing at first, but finding a little extra reason to stick at something can make all the difference, especially when you're starting out. When I'm in a rut, I give myself a challenge for 28 days and it just shifts my attitude and motivation, and ensures I make myself accountable to someone.

HOW TO USE THIS BOOK

I'd love you to use this book in a number of different ways

For those of you in the Transform Phase, I'd like my recipes to show you how easily you can Eat Beautifully, and to help you to achieve fabulous Lean for Life results.

By eating three main meals and two snacks each day you'll stay in the middle of the inner circle and, in combination with the other three pillars (see page 9), you will achieve results that will amaze you. My recipes are all designed to be 'Mr P proof': if my husband can cook them then, seriously, anyone can.

For readers who are in the Lifestyle Phase, these all-new recipes will be a great addition to your repertoire, with lots of fresh options to try. This is one of the ways in which our Method is so different: the recipes reflect the style in which you will eat forever, and not simply when you're trying to lose weight or reach a new goal. Once you're at goal, you simply eat this way most of the time, say 70–80 per cent depending on how active you are. So, long-term, you still eat whatever it is that floats your boat, just in moderation.

This flexibility is key to making Lean for Life a permanent lifestyle change that works for everyone. I want you to try new combinations and make the dishes work for you and your tastes. So if you're a vegetarian, don't like peanuts, or find eggs hard to stomach first thing, develop new combinations based on the foods you do like. Look out for these symbols too: (Vg) denotes vegan recipes and (V) denotes vegetarian ones.

You'll find recipes throughout that can be cooked in many ways: a simple frittata can be adapted to make three deliciously different meals, for example. You'll also learn to 'build' recipes for yourself, playing with new flavour combinations along the way. You'll see each food type as a building block; each piece interchangeable. So as our Method becomes second nature, you can start to develop new recipes and combinations for yourself. The possibilities are endless.

Finally, I want this book to work for your whole family and that's why I've included the Extra Energy Sides and Good Enough for Guests sections. They give another level of flexibility to the book and, I hope, show you just how flexible our Method can be. My family eats this way and the last thing I want is for you to be cooking three meals for five people.

My hope is that my cookbook explains the foundations of Eating Beautifully, provides the inspiration to become Lean for Life and provides the lasting knowledge for you to adapt our Method to suit your needs, whatever life throws your way.

If my husband can cook them then anyone can

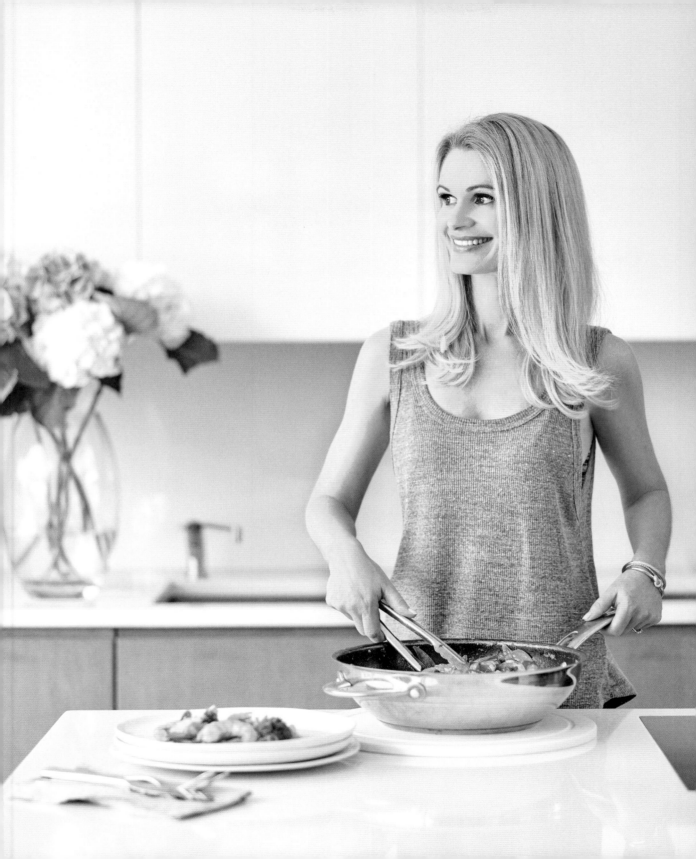

ONE COOKBOOK; ENDLESS RECIPE COMBINATIONS

When I came to write a cookbook, it was important to me that the recipes were precise and simple but not obsessive in matching each recipe with the exact macronutrient profile. This is diet mentality but it is important that you understand the principles, for two reasons:

★ **Firstly,** once you've grasped how and why each recipe is structured the way that it is, you'll be throwing together your own concoctions in no time. And that means endless recipes at your fingertips for life. I want you to be able to look at any recipe or meal you come across anywhere and instantly know how you can adapt it to our Method.

★ **Secondly,** if you are armed with the knowledge to create your own recipes, then it will boost your results, your willpower and will manage your appetite. You mentally commit to it because it makes total sense.

There are more than 140 recipes in this cookbook, but by using the principles to make your own creative adaptations, you can easily fill the years ahead with tasty, healthy meals. Here's how…

How to build a meal

Each Louise Parker Method meal and snack contains a source of protein, some low-GI carbohydrate, a little healthy fat and fibre. We don't eliminate any food group, although we do keep carbohydrates on the lower side.

During the Transform phase, when you're dropping body fat, we strike a careful balance of having enough fuel for your workouts (and to stay healthy and sane), without any excess energy that your body will use as fuel rather than the fat we want to target.

The recipes in this book are here to inspire you, but not confine you. Play around with the dishes while sticking to the principles, and think of 'building' your meals and snacks with food groups as building blocks. If there are any ingredients in a dish you don't love, or can't eat, simply swap them out for something else.

At every meal or snack, the first question to ask yourself is: 'Where is the protein?'. Proteins are the building blocks of your body and an essential element for optimum health, fat loss and muscle preservation. If you don't fancy the protein in a particular recipe you can change it for another, but you do need to include a good portion of protein. For example, swap out the chicken for tofu or eggs if you're a veggie or lobster if you're loaded. You get the idea. Just keep the quantities the same.

Next, think about the lower-GI carbs, which will mainly come from veggies, fruits and high-fibre, low-GI grain-based foods such as oatcakes, oatbran and wholemeal bread. Any of these can be swapped around, and I want you to try new combinations.

Finally, look to add a little portion of good fats. There are a number of natural sources for this, whether it's nuts or seeds, oils in dressings or from fish or eggs… and, of course, that Instagram hero of our age: the avocado. Remember that with certain proteins such as oily fish, eggs, nuts and seeds you'll also be getting a good portion of healthy fats, so you should ease off a little with any additional fats you add in these cases.

I've included Extra Energy Sides (see pages 172–81) – veggies you should ideally avoid during your Transform phase. Once you reach your goal, you can also introduce these a few times a week if you fancy. This section is to inspire you to cook deliciously nutritious sides to allow your family and friends a little extra energy if they need it, without having to cook totally different meals.

I loathe counting calories, which is why I focus instead on portions in my recipes, as these are so much easier to stick to day-to-day. However, do remember that portion size matters. Too much of a good thing – especially extra proteins and fats – will not help you to lose body fat. Every recipe in my books is calibrated to ensure that you are eating a beautiful balance of everything your body needs, while still allowing you to drop body fat.

As the seasons change, and with a little creativity, my recipes will provide you with thousands of options all year round. Do keep changing your kitchen repertoire and experimenting with new flavour combinations, herbs and spices. Just make sure that, as you swap ingredients, you stick to like-for-like portions.

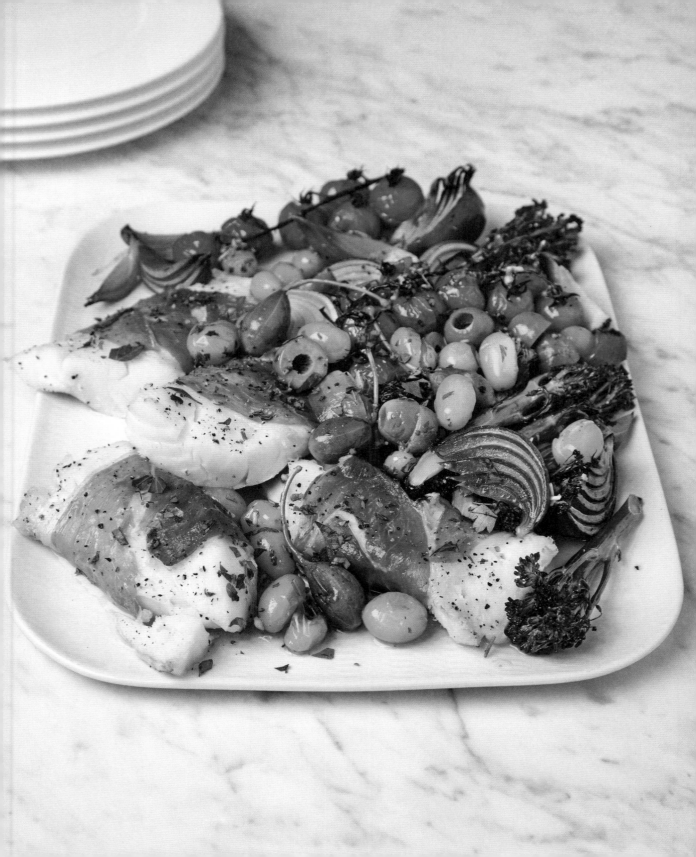

EATING BEAUTIFULLY

1 LOVE FLAVOUR

2 PORTIONS AND CALORIES DO MATTER

3 EAT THREE MEALS AND TWO SNACKS PER DAY

4 ALWAYS BALANCE YOUR FOOD GROUPS

5 SIP, SIP, SIP 2-3 LITRES A DAY – HALF BY LUNCHTIME, HALF BY SUPPERTIME

How to eat with celebration and beauty

★ **Lay the table with a little effort.** It makes each meal just that bit more special.

★ **Invest in lovely tableware, linen napkins and good quality glasses.**

★ **Sofa suppers are real life,** so add a lovely tray and a linen napkin and you've gone from slob to snazzy.

★ **Don't eat out of Tupperware.** Plate up. It'll only take a second and I promise the food will taste better and seem more like a meal.

★ **Just take an extra minute plating up.** Garnish well and plate up as you would for someone special. Fresh herbs and a wedge of lemon is often all it takes.

★ **Never eat standing up.** You'll drop a dress size stopping this habit alone.

★ **Don't eat while walking down the street.** You will bump straight into your ex-boyfriend but, more importantly, you'll forget you've eaten at all.

★ **Do not pick.** Put what you're eating on a plate and know you're eating it. It's too easy to forget you ate 500 fish fingers over the year off your kids' plates.

EATING OUT LEAN
– A GUIDE TO RESTAURANTS

Switching your mindset from 'diet' to 'lifestyle change' is a key component of Lean for Life. So, to fully embrace your new lifestyle, you need to learn to eat lean on the go. It may make sense to avoid the odd social occasion when you're starting your transformation, however, think of Eating Out Lean as a life skill that you're going to master as one of the many benefits of our Method. The beauty is that it's usually really easy, especially once you understand the building blocks of Eating Beautifully.

Eating out on my programme is to be encouraged; it's part of life and there's no reason why you can't follow our Method in just about any restaurant. Some of my clients eat out twice a day due to the nature of their jobs, and in many ways that familiarity makes ordering off piste easier. You just need to learn some simple tricks to navigate a menu.

Here's what you do:

Most restaurants will offer something 'on Method'. French, English, Italian and American are probably the simplest options, as typically they will offer a grilled fish or meat dish, but just about any cuisine will have something for you.

Order like a New Yorker. What I do is scan the proteins on offer and ignore what it comes with. If I want sea bass – but with something that's paired with the steak on the menu – I simply tell the waiter how I'd like it. No menu is set in stone.

Think fine dining whatever the restaurant. Portion control matters. Eating mindfully matters. So slow everything down and enjoy the ceremony of your meal.

Sip first. Always start with a glass of water. It's a really simple way to distinguish thirst from hunger.

If you're having a three-course meal with friends, go for a protein-based starter and main, and skip the bread and pud. I know that's the hardest part for me, but it's a temporary situation. Once you're at goal, you can have the bread, the wine and a little dessert.

Damage control is a victory. Sometimes there are no totally 'on plan' choices, or your host is only serving carbonara. If so, be gracious, enjoy your food and make the best choices you can. Think about eating more veg and less of the carbonara and manage your portions. If before you'd have had a second helping and more, then this is progress.

Remember the dance. It's not a disaster if you step out of the circle. Don't be hard on yourself, simply step back in as soon as you can. Don't look back.

Balance your day. If you know you're likely to have a heavier dinner because you're eating out, opt for a lighter lunch, or even just eat an extra snack instead of lunch. Just don't cut back too much, or your blood sugars will drop and all bets are off.

Be confident. You can totally do this. And what's more, you'll love how you feel when you learn how to eat out with control and in a beautifully lean way.

Remember the dance. It's not a disaster if you step out of the circle

	Monday	Tuesday	Wednesday
BREAKFAST	Paul's Carrot Cake Bircher	Chocolate & Raspberry Porridge	Salmon Tartine with Lemon Cream
SNACK	Chocolate Cinnamon Almonds	Roast Pepper Hummus	Chocolate Cinnamon Almonds
LUNCH	My Favourite Tabbouleh	Roquefort, Pear & Chicory Salad	Brocolli, Butter Bean & Pistachio Soup
SNACK	Roast Pepper Hummus	Seedy Strawbs	Seedy Strawbs
DINNER	Catanina Cod Tray Bake	Grumpa's Creamy Courgette Dhal	Ratatouille with Baked Eggs & Goats' Cheese

Thursday	Friday	Saturday	Sunday

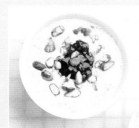

Strawberry Ripple Bircher

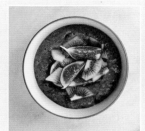

Purple Porridge

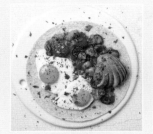

Ale's Huevos Rancheros

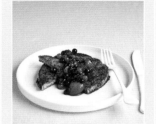

Chocolate French Toast

Winter Nuts

Seedy Strawbs

El Verde Hummus

Ras El Hanout Roasted Chickpeas

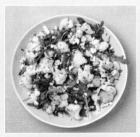

Cauliflower & Feta

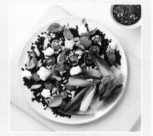

Black & White Beluga Salad

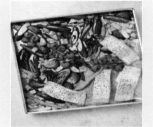

Warm Winter Roast

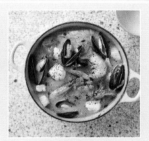

My Seafood Bouillabaisse

Vanilla & Almond Smoothie Bowl

Winter Nuts

Double Deckers

El Verde Hummus

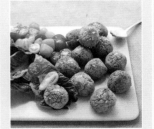

Double Bean Burger Balls

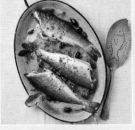

Whole Roasted Sea Bass

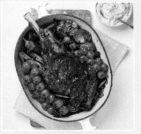

Slow-roast Moroccan Lamb

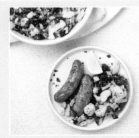

Sophie's Sausages & Smashing Beans

MY LEAN FOR LIFE KITCHEN

I really put effort into creating the right physical environment to allow me to think positively. Our surroundings affect our mood so much. I love design and art and beautiful things, and always have done. Even at boarding school, I had the neatest bedside table and surrounded myself with just a few lovely things that reminded me of home. Today, when my home, office, car and kitchen cupboards are in order, everything is just easy-to-find and pleasing on the eye… and the busy life I lead feels so much less chaotic. It just lifts my mood. OK, I am a neat freak.

I pay particular attention to my kitchen, as it's central to our daily family life. Space is tight, too, and so I'm conscious of only keeping things that are beautiful, practical and used almost daily.

★ **Spring clean year round.** If you stay on top of it, it's never more than a couple of hours' work. Every month I whizz through the kitchen, tunes on, and clear out the cupboards and drawers and rearrange a few things, even if it's just throwing in a new plant or swapping over some of the genius artwork the girls bring home from school. I like my kitchen to be clutter-free, practical, but also beautiful to walk into on a grey Wednesday morning.

* **Organization is obvious.** I know, but this is key, and especially if you have a small kitchen like mine. I've got a jar fetish, but I really like to be able to open up a cupboard and see all my herbs, spices and dried foods in full view. If I can see it, then I will cook with it and it encourages me to use so many more herbs and spices than I would if they were crammed at the back of a shelf, covered in dust. If everything is in jars and nice containers, you can just throw a few ingredients on the table at mealtimes so everyone can customize their meals themselves. It's a great way to get faddy children to try new things.

* **Create a beautiful space.** Do what it takes to make your kitchen a place you want to be. It doesn't need to cost a penny, but just some thoughtful rearranging can really create an environment that you'll want to spend more time in… at the same time it allows you to get out of it more quickly – because it's organized – on the days when you only want to flop and relax on the sofa.

Here are some of my personal kitchen essentials:

I don't go in for heaps of kitchen gadgets. I want everything I own to perform a multitude of tasks, and less is always more. I do own a waffle maker, bread maker, ice-cream maker, panini press and even a mini chocolate fountain, but I store the things I rarely use high up and out of the way. These are the things that never gather dust:

Vitamix. It's a big investment but, for me, it's the best professional blender by a long shot. It's no wonder every Michelin-starred kitchen has a professional blender, as it actually intensifies flavour and as an added bonus it's so quick to clean. I am not on commission, but I should be, because I am their greatest fan.

Sharp knives. These make such a difference in terms of speed and are much safer than blunt knives. I keep them in a fabric storage roll and sharpen often.

Chopping boards. I use an ugly plastic board for chicken that I replace regularly and then three or four wooden boards beautiful enough to serve food straight to the table.

Good baking trays and sheets. I use non-stick and replace them whenever they are on sale.

Filtered water taps. I was luckily given a Grohe one that gives you boiling, filtered still, mildly and extra sparkling water. I love not having to buy bottled water, or wait for a kettle to boil, and we all drink so much more water now.

Nespresso machine. Neat, tiny and used daily.

Le Creuset pans. I love the non-stick stainless-steel ones but use the cast-iron ones for casseroles and oven cooking. Invest in a good griddle pan, omelette pan and wok.

Joseph Joseph storage boxes. Functional, easy to stack.

Little bits and bobs. A garlic press, lime zester and Microplane; a spiralizer and a metal steak tenderizer; a wooden lemon squeezer, a veggie peeler, a Masterclass olive oil diffuser which is refillable (get one); a salt pig full of sea salt and – last but not least – seriously good salt and pepper mills.

I keep three preserve bottles of infused oils out on display. Everything looks better in threes: a rosemary and thyme; a hot-as-hell chilli; and a roasted garlic and herbes de Provence. Use mild olive oil as the base.

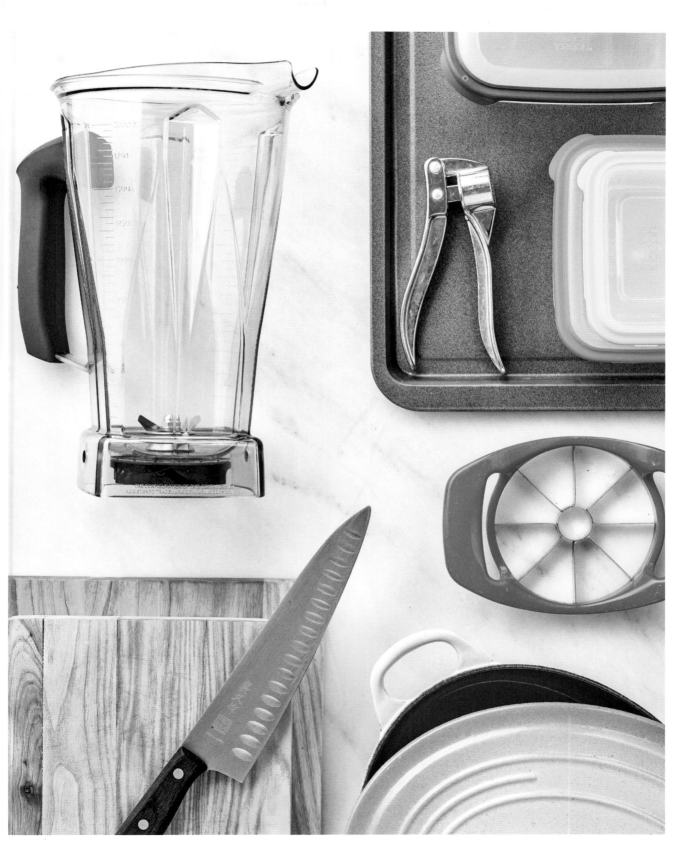

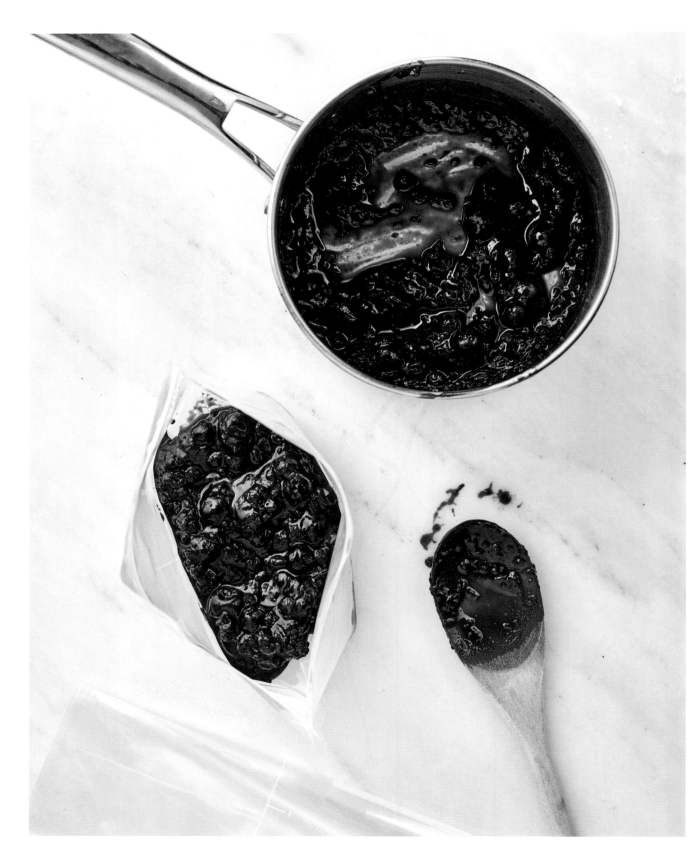

Organization – lean bodies come prepared

They just do. You simply can't leave your food choices down to chance and hope to get lucky and change your body and your lifestyle. Having said that, you also need to keep things realistic and in perspective. We're creating habits to last forever, not white-knuckling through some 'New Year, New You' diet that fizzles out by February.

I don't want to dedicate a day a week to putting my meals in Tupperware. This kills the joy and celebration of it. I mostly enjoy the 10 minutes spent preparing meals as time to help me switch off and rest, and nothing beats the taste of fresh ingredients. So think about preparing like someone who has a life, rather than turning it into a full-time hobby, or even obsession.

Cook in batches, as and when you can and feel like it. I simply don't have the time or inclination to spend a day doing a big cook-up for the week ahead. It's my idea of hell. Whenever you're making somethinthat freezes well, double or triple up the recipe, so you've got something to snatch out of the freezer in the morning when you need it.

Bits on the side. If you are taking food from home, separate out anything that will make your meal go soggy. A simple way is to wrap items such as tomatoes or cucumbers separately, and always add any dressing just before you eat (so if you are planning to pack up a salad for lunch tomorrow, only dress the bit you're eating today, so you can pack the undressed salad and dressing separately for the next day). Keep a stash of salt, pepper, olive oil, and condiments with you at work so you don't even need to take dressing with you each day.

Non-stick, dishwasher-safe pans. Sometimes it's not the preparation but the cleaning up that takes the most time. Buying some new pans and making sure everything is dishwasher-safe, so you don't have to spend hours scrubbing, is an incredibly simple way to save valuable time. I buy nothing that does not go in a dishwasher, except special wine glasses.

Buy well. If you stock up your kitchen with lean ingredients, it's the easiest way to make sure you always eat lean meals. If you can, arrange for weekly food deliveries to save time. If weekly deliveries won't work for your schedule, then always have some fresh items with a longer shelf life just in case. For me, these are frozen prawns, feta and goats' cheeses, tofu, frozen vegetables and eggs. This way if you run out of 'fresh' ingredients, you can always throw some store cupboard staples together to create a delicious stir-fry or omelette.

Make sure your pantry is properly stocked. You can always knock up a meal with a good-quality can of tuna, a few capers, a can of beans, seasoning and the odd veggie that is lurking in the salad drawer. I always keep canned tomatoes, lots of varieties of beans, tuna and anchovies. I also keep jars of capers and caperberries and always have packs of ready-cooked lentils for rainy days.

You know how I feel about jars. Keep all your nuts, spices, herbs and seasonings always fully stocked.

Eat the same meal as everyone else in the family. Tweak your meals and make use of my Extra Energy Sides for growing children and husbands, but don't cook 'your food' and 'their food'. You'll lose the plot and it feeds the 'diet mentality'. My kids have to try everything 6 times before they declare they 'don't like it'.

Prepare like someone who has a life, rather than an obsession

1

BREAKFASTS

Breakfast is my favourite meal of the day. It's imperative we make time for it, too, if maintaining a lean body for life is our goal. I know how frenetic mornings can be, and how lost keys and forgotten appointments can turn what was meant to be a blissful family meal into a near meltdown. During the week, it might be the only meal we all have together. I rely on fast, fit food: birchers that soak overnight and can be just spooned up; speedy oatbran porridge; warm toast with nut butters; or berry sauce that can be tossed over yogurt in seconds. If I've got early meetings, I'm often drinking a protein smoothie while applying my mascara. Weekend breakfasts are slower affairs, and the girls join in making pancakes, omelettes and all the other recipes that take just that little bit longer. It's all about finding a routine that works for you and your family, but do try to make it a pleasure and not a rush.

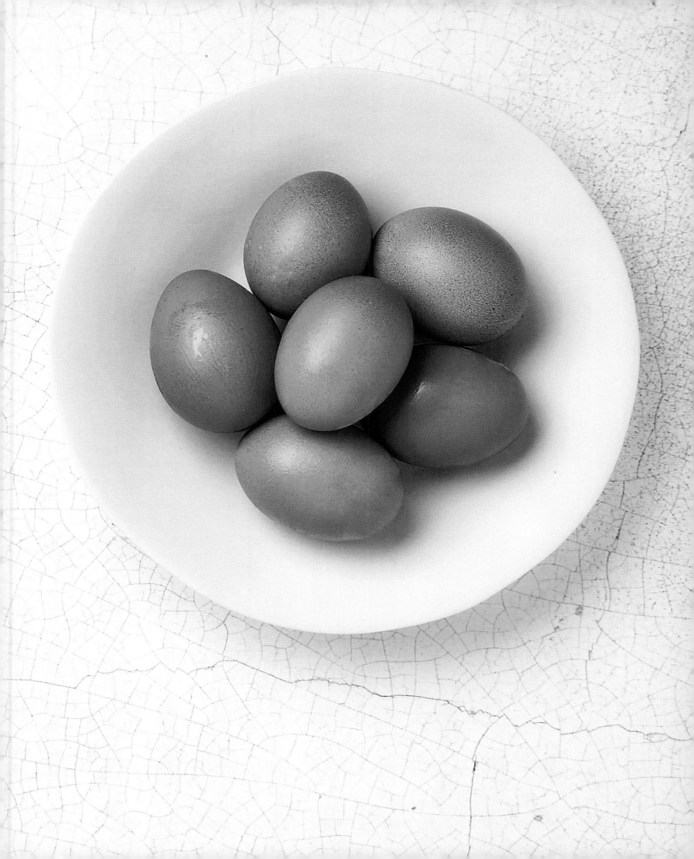

Ale's Huevos Rancheros ⓥ

Serves 4

1 tablespoon rapeseed or other vegetable oil, plus more to fry the eggs

4 red onions, cut into chunks

400g (2 cups) cherry tomatoes, halved

4 jalapeño or other chillies, deseeded if you like less heat, plus more to serve

2 teaspoons sea salt

300ml (scant 1¼ cups) water

8 large eggs

4 wholemeal tortilla wraps

2 ripe avocados, sliced

handful of coriander leaves, chopped

1 lime, quartered

This is a favourite of our Mexican dietician, Alejandra – who is the most fantastic cook – and goes by the saying that everything tastes better with chilli and lime, which I can't argue with. I adore this dish. You can leave out the chilli if you are cooking for younger children; they'll love getting stuck in and a little bit messy.

Heat the rapeseed oil in a frying pan over a medium heat (make sure the frying pan you choose has a lid). Add the onions and sauté for 4 minutes. Add the tomatoes, chilli and salt and stir for 5 minutes.

Pour in the water, pop the lid on and leave to simmer away for 10 minutes.

Pop half the sauce in a blender and whizz, then return the puréed mixture to the rest of the sauce.

Now fry the eggs in a little oil in another frying pan until they are done to your liking. Warm the tortilla wraps in a low oven, or in the frying pan once the eggs are cooked (they only need a few seconds).

Place the eggs and sauce on the warm tortillas, with the sliced avocado. Sprinkle with the coriander and serve with the lime wedges and extra chilli on the side.

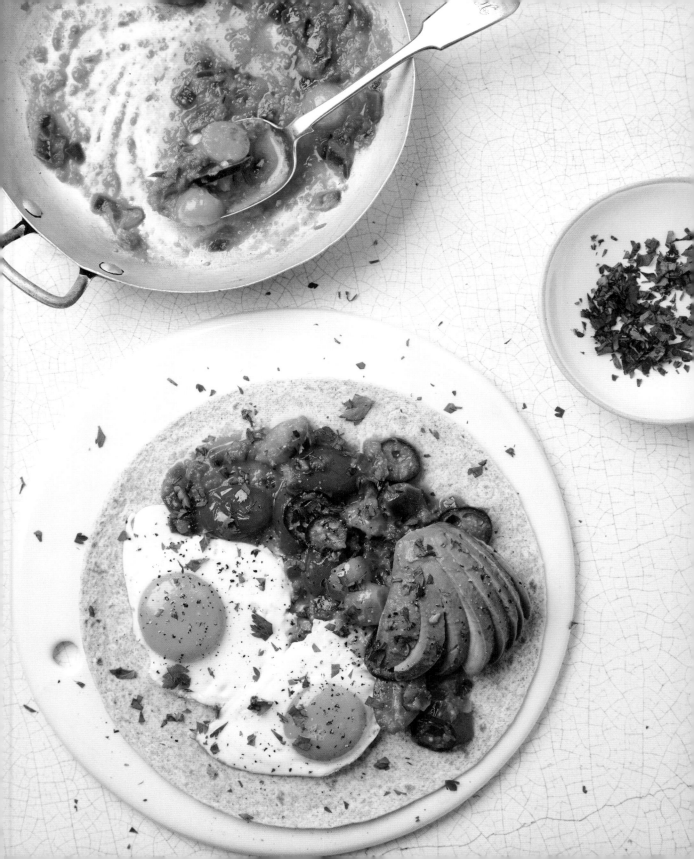

Greco's Coriander Eggs ⓥ

Serves 4

FOR THE EGGS

1 tablespoon groundnut oil

8 eggs

leaves from 1 bunch of coriander,
finely chopped

1 large mild red chilli, chopped
(optional)

1 large mild green chilli, chopped
(optional)

4 wholemeal English muffins, toasted
(lids on for the kids, ½ a muffin per egg
for adults)

a little salted butter, softened

FOR THE SALSA

juice of 2 limes, rolled firmly first to
help release the juice

400g (2 cups) green tomatoes,
deseeded and chopped

1 shallot, finely chopped

1 green apple, finely chopped

2 ripe avocados

handful of flat leaf parsley, chopped

sea salt and black pepper

I love weekends away at the Grecos'. Paul's best friend is a culinary genius and I always come home with new tips and tight jeans. I've tweaked this favourite breakfast (which I believe is Rose Prince's invention) from these visits. Play with different flavourings and remember which ones have the chillies in if you're feeding kids.

Firstly prepare the eggs. Brush a little oil over a ramekin, then line with a large piece of clingfilm. Brush a little more oil on the clingfilm, or the egg will stick to that. Break an egg in, sprinkle with the chopped coriander and chilli, if using, then bring the clingfilm up and twist the top until totally secure. Repeat to wrap all the eggs.

Now your little egg parcels are secure and ready to poach, you can get your salsa ready, which can sit for a while as the lime juice will keep it bright green. Combine the juice of 1 of the limes with the tomatoes, shallot and apple. Dice the avocados and drench with the juice of the other lime. Add to the tomato mixture, taste for seasoning and sprinkle with parsley.

Bring a saucepan of water to a rolling boil. Now dunk the wrapped eggs into the boiling water with a slotted spoon – I cook 2 at a time – and simmer for 3 minutes. Now drop into a bowl of ice-cold water, which will make it easier to unwrap, just for a few seconds. Repeat to poach all the eggs.

Toast the muffins and scrape with a bit of butter.

Unwrap 2 eggs on to each muffin and serve with the salsa.

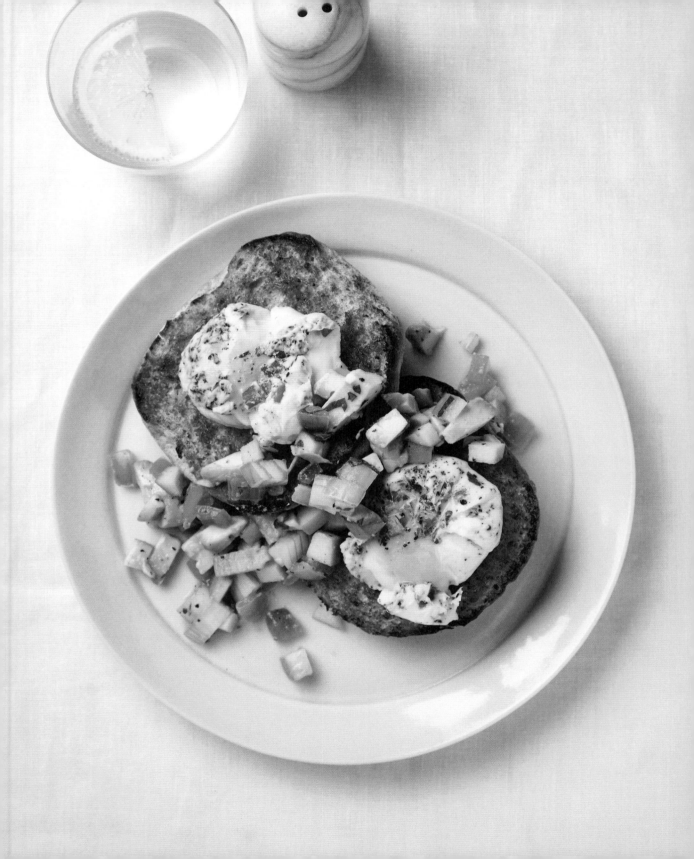

BIRCHER 6 WAYS

I know, I know, more Bircher. But I just adore it because you can make it the night before, in two minutes flat, and adapt it with so many different fruits and flavours. It's also abundant in protein, fibre and goodness and is low-GI – the perfect fit, fast breakfast.

① Classic Vanilla (V)

Serves 4

500g (2 cups) low-fat Greek yogurt

4 heaped tablespoons oatbran (80g/2¾oz)

75ml (⅓ cup) semi-skimmed (1 or 2%) milk, plus more if needed

½ teaspoon vanilla paste

stevia, to taste (add this in the morning and adjust)

Combine all the ingredients except the stevia together thoroughly and place in the fridge overnight to soak. In the morning, taste and add the stevia. You can also adjust the consistency by adding more milk, if you like.

② Vanilla Vegan (Vg)

Serves 4

500g (2 cups) unsweetened soya yogurt

4 heaped tablespoons oatbran (80g/2¾oz)

½ teaspoon vanilla paste

a little soya milk, if needed

Combine all the ingredients together thoroughly and place in the fridge overnight to soak. In the morning, adjust the consistency by adding soya milk, if you like.

③ CoCo's Coconut (V)

Serves 4

FOR THE BIRCHER

1 quantity of Classic Vanilla or Vanilla Vegan (see left)

4 tablespoons unsweetened desiccated coconut

75ml (⅓ cup) coconut water (Classic Vanilla only), plus more if needed

a little semi-skimmed (1 or 2%) milk, if needed

FOR THE TOPPING

2 tablespoons unsweetened coconut flakes

1 teaspoon poppy seeds

The night before, combine the Classic Vanilla or Vanilla Vegan ingredients and stir in the desiccated coconut. Soak overnight in the fridge.

In the morning, add the stevia, if using, and taste and adjust to your desired consistency with a little milk or a dash more coconut water (the vegan version is less thick, so doesn't require extra liquid).

Toast the coconut flakes in a dry frying pan over a medium heat, until nutty and golden. Sprinkle on top of the Bircher, along with the poppy seeds.

④ Rhubarb Crumble ⓥ

Serves 4

FOR THE BIRCHER

1 quantity of Classic Vanilla or Vanilla Vegan
(see opposite)

FOR THE RHUBARB

8 rhubarb stalks, cut into 2-cm (¾-inch) pieces

50ml (scant ¼ cup) water

juice of 1 orange

½ teaspoon finely grated unwaxed orange zest

1 teaspoon stevia

FOR THE CRUMBLE

1 heaped tablespoon shop-bought low-GI granola

1 tablespoon dehydrated raspberry pieces

1 tablespoon chopped, toasted hazelnuts

Place the rhubarb, water and orange juice in a
saucepan and bring to a simmer for 20 minutes,
until soft and almost sticky. Stir in the orange zest
and sweeten with the stevia, a little at a time, until
you get your desired sweetness. Allow to cool.

Stir together all the ingredients for the crumble.

Serve the rhubarb swirled through the Bircher and
sprinkle with the crumble.

⑤ Paul's Carrot Cake ⓥ

Serves 4

1 quantity of Classic Vanilla or
Vanilla Vegan (see opposite)

2 carrots, finely grated

1 teaspoon ground cinnamon

½ teaspoon ground nutmeg

1 red apple, grated, skin on

a little plant-based milk, if needed

The night before, combine the Classic Vanilla or
Vanilla Vegan ingredients and stir in the carrots,
spices and apple. Soak overnight in the fridge

In the morning, add the stevia, if using. Taste and
adjust to your desired consistency with a little milk
and serve topped with extra carrot and nutmeg,
if desired.

⑥ Strawberry Ripple ⓥ

Serves 4

4 servings of Quick Strawberry Jam (see page 52)

1 quantity of Classic Vanilla Bircher or
Vanilla Vegan Bircher (see opposite)

4 passion fruits

2 tablespoons salted pistachios, chopped

Swirl the strawberry jam through the Bircher and
divide the mixture between 4 bowls. Stir through
the pulp of 1 passion fruit into each bowl and
sprinkle with the pistachios.

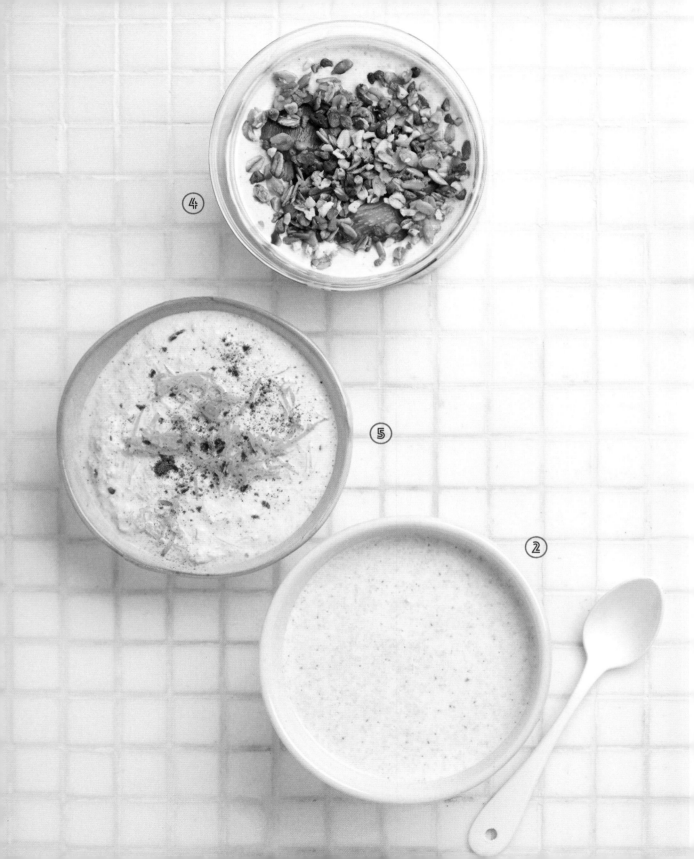

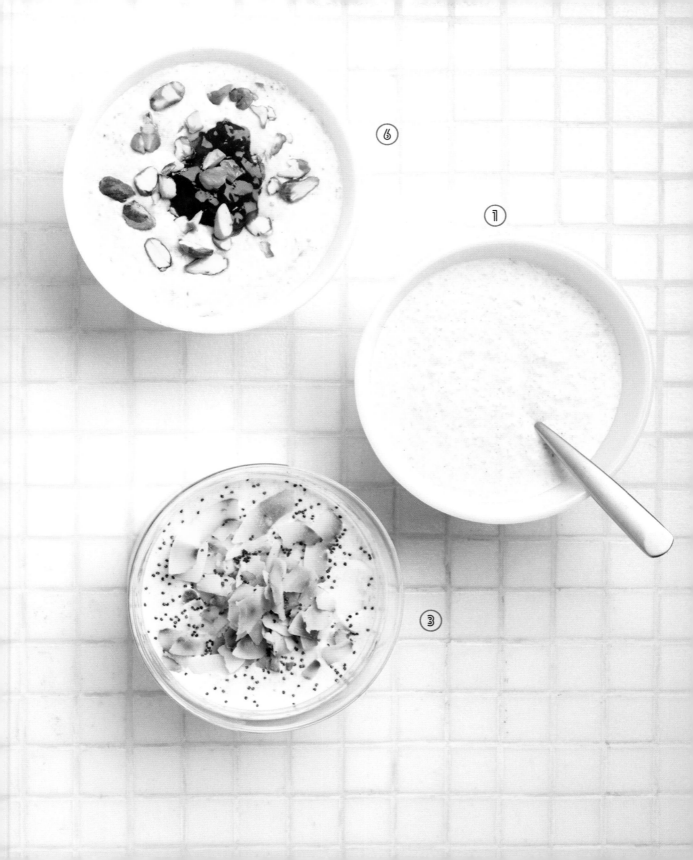

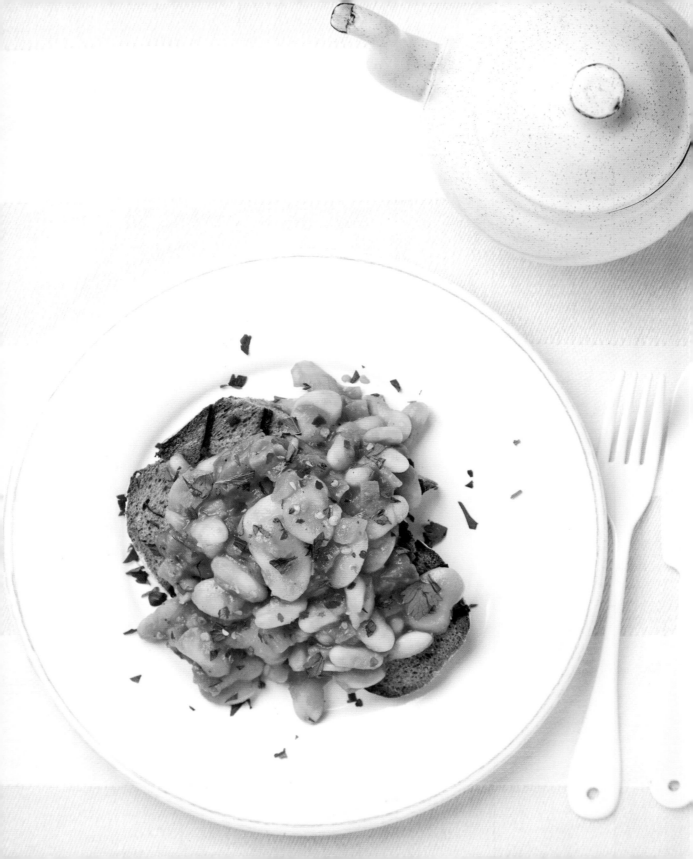

Smoky Beans on Toast (Vg)

Serves 4 (with leftovers)

FOR THE BEANS

1 tablespoon olive oil

1 red onion, finely chopped

1 celery stick, finely chopped

1 carrot, finely chopped

2 teaspoons sweet smoked paprika

1 garlic clove, roughly chopped

1 thyme sprig

400g (14oz) can cannellini beans, drained and rinsed

400g (14oz) can butter beans, drained and rinsed

400g (14oz) can cherry tomatoes

100ml (scant ½ cup) water

1 tablespoon red wine vinegar

sea salt and black pepper

good handful of flat leaf parsley leaves, chopped

chilli flakes, to serve

FOR THE TOAST

4 slices of good wholemeal bread

drizzle of olive oil

1 garlic clove, halved

This is the vegan base of my homemade beans, that are so simple to make and great for batch-cooking. If you don't need this to be veggie, try adding chorizo with the onions instead of the paprika, or vary it with lean bacon and a good dose of herbes de Provence. This recipe works with any beans and is particularly good with chilli and lots of fresh herbs. Play around and find your favourite combination.

Preheat the oven to 160°C/325°F/Gas Mark 3.

Heat the olive oil in a casserole dish over a medium heat. Add the onion, celery and carrot and stir until the onion is translucent. Now add the paprika and garlic and stir for a minute, before throwing in the thyme, both types of beans, the tomatoes and water. Give it all a quick stir, put the lid on and pop it into the oven for 20 minutes (longer cooking will give you drier beans, so this is a matter of taste).

Remove, stir in the red wine vinegar and season to taste.

Now heat up a griddle pan over a really high heat. Brush both sides of the bread with a tiny bit of olive oil and rub the halved garlic clove swiftly across both sides. Grill each side of the toast on the griddle pan until fragrant and stripy.

Serve the beans on the toast and sprinkle with the parsley and chilli flakes.

Salmon Tartine with Lemon Cream

Serves 1

50g (¼ cup) reduced-fat
cream cheese

2 tablespoons 0% Greek yogurt

1 teaspoon finely grated unwaxed
lemon zest

1 slice of good wholemeal bread

50g (2oz) sliced smoked salmon

sea salt and black pepper

pinch of chilli flakes (optional)

1 teaspoon chopped flat leaf
parsley leaves

4 caperberries, halved, or 12 capers

½ lemon, cut into wedges

A tartine makes a great breakfast or brunch with friends and can easily be made ahead. In the summer you can grill the toast outside on a barbecue and serve it with buffalo mozzarella and roasted red peppers dressed in balsamic vinegar and capers, seasoned well with crunchy sea salt. Another family favourite is to simply toast the bread, brush it with a teaspoon of good bought tapenade, then add rocket leaves, prosciutto slices and cherry tomatoes. The possibilities are endless, just don't forget the protein and a good couple of portions of veggies.

In a bowl, using a fork, mix together the cream cheese, yogurt and lemon zest. Toast the bread – or griddle it on a very hot griddle pan for a smoky flavour, if you prefer – and spread thickly with the cream cheese mixture.

Arrange the smoked salmon on top. Season to taste, using salt and pepper or chilli and serve sprinkled with parsley and with lemon wedges and caperberries or capers on the side.

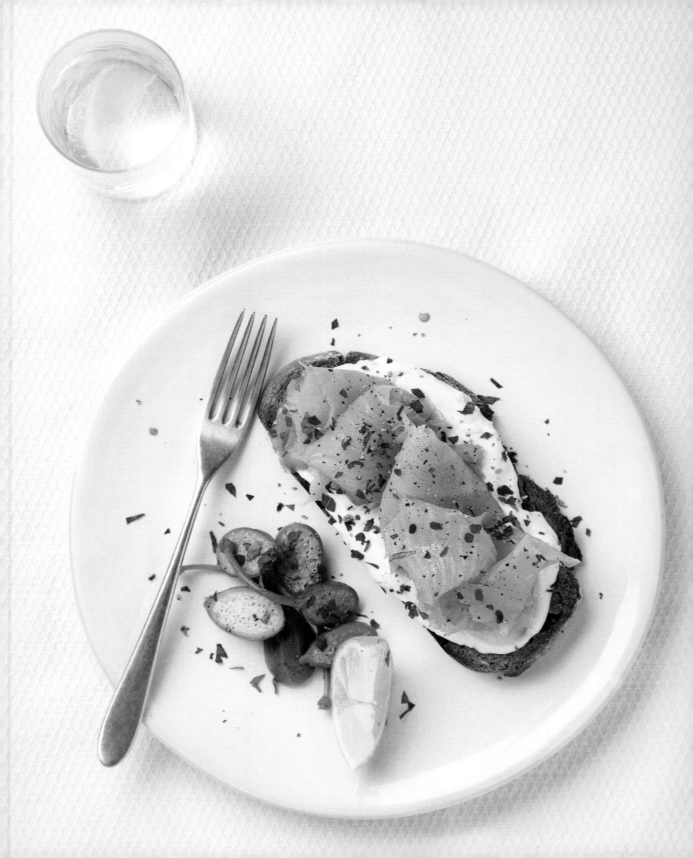

Smoked Bacon Rolls with Easy Tomato Chutney

Serves 4

FOR THE CHUTNEY

1 tablespoon olive oil

2 shallots, finely chopped

150g (¾ cup) red cherry tomatoes, halved

150g (¾ cup) yellow cherry tomatoes, left whole

1 garlic clove, chopped

1 teaspoon good balsamic vinegar

pinch of stevia (optional)

sea salt and black pepper

FOR THE ROLLS

8 lean bacon rashers, ideally smoked

4 small wholemeal rolls

a little salted butter, softened

8 Baby Gem lettuce leaves

4 thick slices of beef tomato

This is a Sunday morning favourite of ours, often eaten as a 'second breakfast' after an active morning playing in the park. Chose the best bacon you can afford and, once grilled, cut off the visible fat. The relish keeps for a good few days in the fridge, and you can tweak it in so many ways: try capers and basil leaves stirred through once cooked, or chop in some chilli and coriander leaves for the grown-ups. Canned cherry tomatoes work perfectly well, too.

Start with the chutney. Choose a large non-stick frying pan (using non-stick allows you to use less oil) and place over a medium heat with the oil. Add the shallots and cook until translucent but not browned. Throw in the tomatoes and reduce the heat to low. Add the garlic and seasoning and allow it to simmer until nicely reduced and a bit gooey, which will take about 10 minutes.

Meanwhile, grill the bacon and cut the rolls in half. Spread each roll with a scraping of butter on each side (the softer the better) and add the lettuce and a big fat slice of tomato.

Now add a splash of balsamic vinegar to the tomatoes to give them that chutney twang. Check the seasoning; depending on how ripe and sweet the tomatoes are, you might want to add a tiny – and I mean tiny – pinch of stevia.

Fill the rolls with the bacon and a good dollop of chutney and get messy.

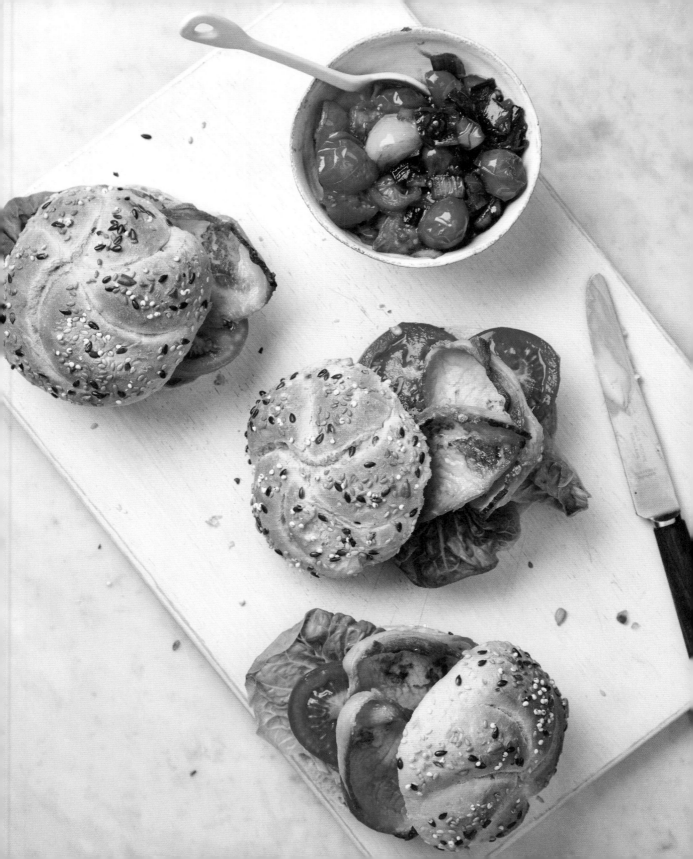

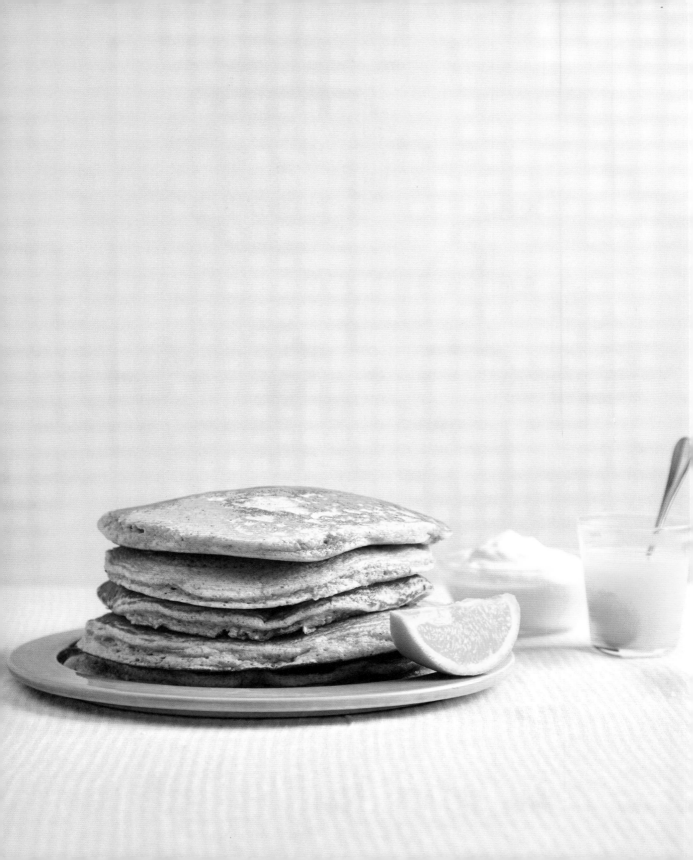

Orange Pancakes with Lemon Drizzle & Ricotta Cream ⓥ

Serves 4

FOR THE PANCAKES

4 tablespoons oatbran

4 tablespoons wholemeal flour

4 tablespoons dried skimmed milk

8 tablespoons soya milk

4 large eggs

1 teaspoon vanilla paste

½ teaspoon stevia

1 heaped teaspoon baking powder

½ teaspoon finely grated unwaxed orange zest

4 teaspoons unsalted butter

FOR THE DRIZZLE

juice of 2 lemons

juice of 1 orange, 1 tablespoon reserved for the ricotta cream

stevia, to taste

FOR THE RICOTTA CREAM

100g (½ cup) ricotta cheese

200g (¾ cup) Greek yogurt

1 tablespoon orange juice

½ teaspoon finely grated unwaxed orange zest

My protein-rich pancakes can be served with endless sugar-free toppings. Try my homemade quick strawberry jam, or hot summer berry vitality sauce (see pages 52 and 54), or simply add 1 tablespoon of cocoa powder and a little extra stevia into the batter mixture for a chocolate pancake, which is delicious spread with my chocolate hazlenut butter (see page 60) and sprinkled with toasted hazelnut pieces.

Combine the oatbran, flour and dried milk in a blender, then add the soya milk, eggs, vanilla paste, stevia and baking powder. Blend for 30 seconds until everything is combined, being careful not to over-process to keep the pancakes light. Now stir in the orange zest (don't blend this into the mix).

Melt the butter in a non-stick frying pan over a medium heat. Add a generous tablespoon of the batter to form each pancake. When the mixture forms little bubbles on the surface, they are good to flip.

Meanwhile, prepare the drizzle by heating the lemon and orange juices until they reduce slightly. Taste and add stevia if you wish.

Prepare the ricotta cream by mixing together the ricotta and yogurt with the orange juice and zest.

Serve the pancakes, with a little drizzle and the ricotta cream.

PORRIDGE 5 WAYS

I always use pure oatbran as it has 50 per cent more fibre, more protein, vitamins and minerals than normal oats. So it will fill you up, nourish you and reduce cholesterol. I make sure I have at least 2 tablespoons a day. Play around with the consistency to suit your taste and try soya milk or lactose-free milk if you're lactose intolerant. Avoid almond and rice milk though as these are higher in sugar. Add more oats if you feel you need a bigger portion.

① Classic Vanilla (Vg)

Serves 4

8 heaped tablespoons oatbran (160g/5¾oz)

750ml (3 cups) soya milk, plus more if needed

2 teaspoons vanilla paste

couple of pinches of sea salt, to taste

Combine the oatbran with the milk, vanilla and salt in a saucepan.

Place over a medium heat and bring to a simmer for 2 minutes until the porridge bubbles and turns a creamy consistency.

Adjust to your preferred consistency with a dash more milk, or use less to start with if you prefer it a bit thicker.

② Spiced Blackberry & Apple (Vg)

Serves 4

1 quantity Classic Vanilla oatbran porridge (see left)

2 red apples, skin on, cut into cubes

½ teaspoon ground cinnamon

½ teaspoon ground nutmeg

150g (1 cup) blackberries

Prepare the porridge, using just 500ml (2 cups) of milk and including the apples, cinnamon and nutmeg at the start. Only when the porridge is done, add the blackberries, giving them a good stir through. Depending on how juicy the apples are, check the consistency and add more milk until you reach a texture you like.

③ Chocolate & Raspberry Ⓥ

Serves 4

2 tablespoons cocoa powder

1 tablespoon hot water

2 good tablespoons hazelnut butter

1 quantity Classic Vanilla oatbran porridge
(see opposite)

4 teaspoons dried raspberry pieces

4 pinches of flavourless popping candy (optional)

Mix the cocoa powder thoroughly into the hot water to make a paste, then combine with the hazelnut butter (you can do this in a big batch; it's great as a sugar-free alternative to chocolate hazelnut spread). Swirl into the hot porridge. Top with the raspberry pieces and a pinch of popping candy, if liked, just before serving.

④ Purple Porridge Ⓥg

Serves 4

1 quantity Classic Vanilla oatbran porridge
(see opposite)

150g (1 scant cup) frozen blueberries

4 fresh figs, sliced

1 kiwifruit, peeled and sliced

Prepare the porridge, adding the blueberries as it starts to cook so that they pop and bleed their purple colour into the porridge. Decorate with slices of fig and kiwifruit.

⑤ Coconut, Cashew & Banana Ⓥg

Serves 4

1 quantity Classic Vanilla oatbran porridge
(see opposite)

4 tablespoons unsweetened desiccated coconut

2 bananas, sliced

2 good tablespoons cashew nut butter

a few unsweetened, toasted coconut flakes, to serve

Prepare the porridge, adding in the desiccated coconut at the start. After 90 seconds, pop in the banana if you don't mind little lumps, or include it at the start to please little people who are suspicious of lumps. You can combine the cashew butter early on, too, or swirl it on top when it's piping hot. As your porridge is cooking, toast the coconut flakes in a dry frying pan just until they start to turn golden. Sprinkle on top of your breakfast bowl.

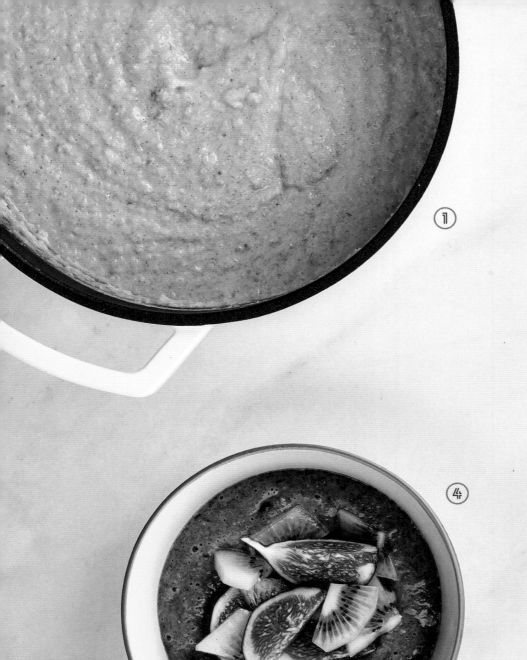

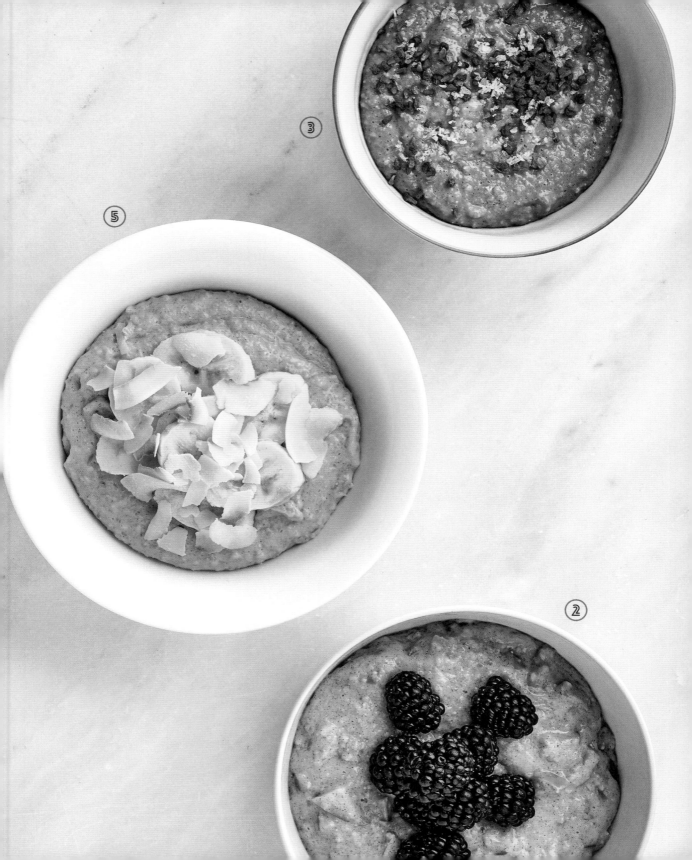

Grilled Ricotta ⓥ

Fabulous for a winter breakfast, on the sofa, fire on.

Serves 4

FOR THE QUICK STRAWBERRY JAM

400g (2 cups) ripe or frozen strawberries, hulled

stevia, to taste (optional)

FOR THE RICOTTA

300g (1¼ cups) ricotta cheese

½ teaspoon finely grated unwaxed lemon zest, plus more to serve

½ teaspoon vanilla paste

4 slices of walnut bread

handful of walnuts

a few mint sprigs, to serve

Start with the jam. Cook the strawberries in a saucepan over a medium heat, stirring until the berries reduce to a good thick consistency. Taste and sweeten with stevia, if desired.

Preheat the grill to medium. Mix together the ricotta, lemon zest and vanilla paste. Toast the walnut bread. Spread the ricotta evenly over the pieces of toast. Pop under the grill, and grill until the ricotta begins to brown; this should take about 2 minutes.

Meanwhile, put the walnuts in a dry frying pan over a medium heat and toast, stirring, just until they darken slightly and smell fragrant. Tip on to a plate to stop the cooking.

Serve the ricotta toast with the strawberry jam, either hot or cooled. Sprinkle with the toasted walnuts and lemon zest and mint sprigs.

Baked Pears ⓥ

The smell of baked fruit is just divine. Friends visiting for brunch will comment on the delicious aroma the moment they walk through the door.

Serves 4

FOR THE PEARS

6 walnuts

sea salt

4 pears, cored and halved

4 teeny knobs (pats) of unsalted butter

pinch of ground nutmeg

pinch of ground cinnamon

FOR THE VANILLA POT

100g (⅓ cup) low-fat Greek yogurt

50g (¼ cup) ricotta cheese

½ teaspoon vanilla paste

pinch of stevia, to taste

Preheat the oven to 200°C/400°F/Gas Mark 6.

Put the walnuts in a dry frying pan over a medium heat and stir until they darken and smell toasty. Tip on to a plate and sprinkle with sea salt. When they are cool, chop them roughly.

Place the pears cut side up on a large sheet of foil, with a tiny knob of butter on each. Sprinkle evenly with the spices and bake in the middle of the oven for 20–30 minutes, or until golden.

Mix together the yogurt, ricotta and vanilla and taste. Add stevia if you would like the mixture a little sweeter. Spoon into 4 ramekins or small bowls.

Serve the warm pears with the vanilla pots, sprinkling the pears with the toasted walnuts.

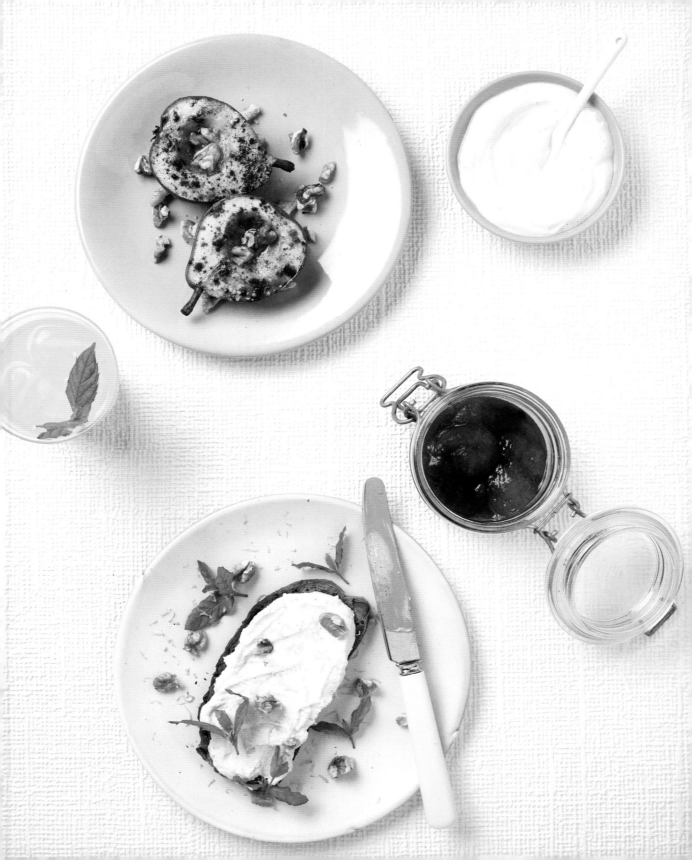

Chocolate French Toast with Vitality Sauce ⓥ

Serves 4

FOR THE VITALITY SAUCE

300g (2 cups) frozen summer berries

1 teaspoon stevia

squeeze of lemon juice

FOR THE FRENCH TOAST

4 large eggs

2 tablespoons milk

½ teaspoon ground cinnamon

1–2 teaspoons cocoa powder

½–1 teaspoon stevia

4 pieces of wholemeal bread, crusts on, each cut into 2 triangles

4 tiny knobs (pats) of unsalted butter

I often make a vanilla version of this toast and serve it with grilled peaches, plums, nectarines or figs, adding a little dollop of my ricotta cream (see page 202). For a savoury version, simply leave out the stevia and vanilla and serve hot with a slice of Gruyère cheese and ham hock and some roasted tomatoes with basil.

First make the sauce. Always use frozen berries, as they're available all year round and are packed full of vitamins. Simply throw the frozen berries in a pan, add the stevia and lemon juice, place over a medium heat and leave to simmer away for 3–5 minutes until it has reduced a little. Set aside to cool slightly.

Now take a bowl and whisk together the eggs, milk, cinnamon, cocoa and stevia. Pour into a large flat dish and, in batches, soak each piece of bread for at least 1 minute on each side.

Place a non-stick frying pan over a medium heat, add a little knob of butter and swirl until the pan is coated in melted butter, then fry each slice on both sides until nicely browned and fluffy.

Serve the French toast with a generous helping of the vitality sauce spooned over the top.

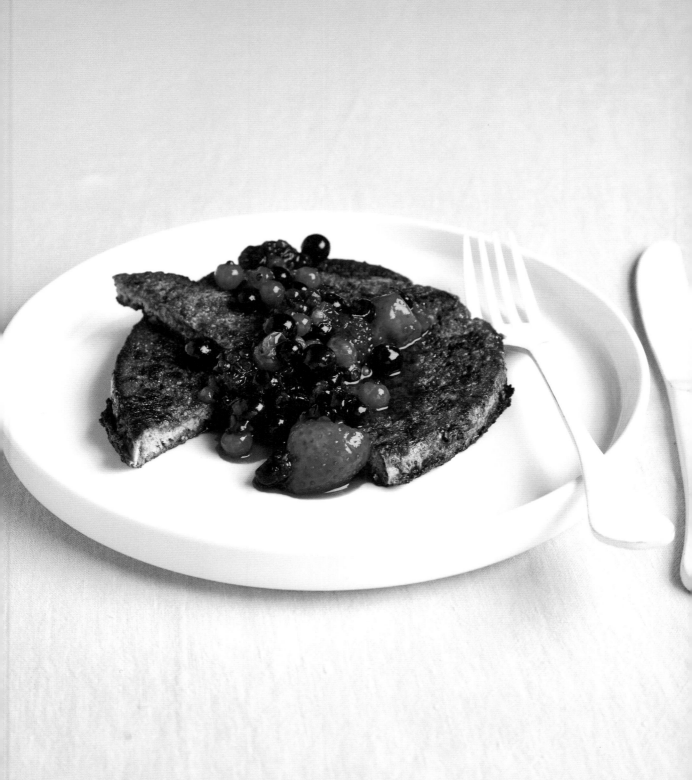

2

SNACKS

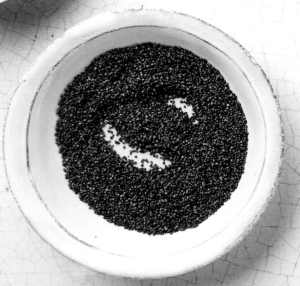

One of the primary principles of Eating Beautifully (see page 22) is the spacing out of your meals. It helps stabilize hormones and blood sugar levels, which gives your willpower the biggest helping hand. It's about preventing you feeling hungry (though finding yourself a little peckish before meals is normal), so that you can always make wise food choices. The secret is preparation: the night before, think about your day ahead. Where will you be? Where could you get caught out without a meal or snack? Carry portable snacks for busy days at work (nuts and a piece of fruit are brilliantly simple), and then on days you work from home – or over the weekend – you can afford to give the more time-consuming recipes in this section a go. But mix it up and don't get bored. You simply have to snack if you want the best results, so please don't overlook this. It's about eating delicately throughout the day. If you get hungry, all bets are off and you're going to steal sweets off children in the street.

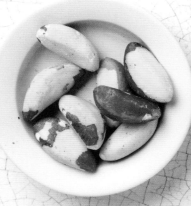

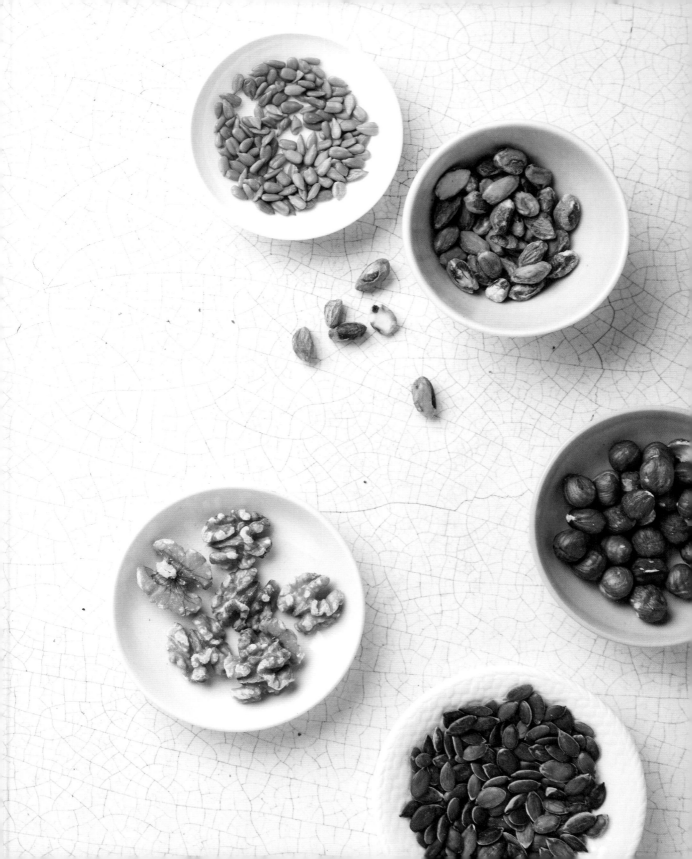

MINI PROTEIN SOUFFLÉS

These are fabulous as snacks and will keep in an airtight container in the fridge for a good couple of days. Do experiment with flavours and different herbs and cheeses. You can bake them in muffin trays, muffin cases or in a sheet pan and cut into squares.

① Stilton & Pea ⓥ

Makes 12

12 eggs, separated

200g (7oz) Stilton

sea salt and black pepper

150g (1 generous cup) frozen peas, defrosted

Preheat the oven to 200°C/400°F/Gas Mark 6.

Whisk the egg whites until they are firm.

Now give the egg yolks a good whisk, crumble in the stilton and season. Do not whisk, but give it a little stir, then fold the egg whites into the egg yolk mixture. Divide the peas between the 12 holes of a muffin tray and then top with the egg mixture.

Place in the centre of the oven and bake for 10 minutes, taking care not to open the oven. Open the door and allow the soufflés to cool a little in the oven, before allowing them to cool fully at room temperature.

② Feta & Spinach ⓥ

Makes 12

200g (7oz) frozen spinach

½ teaspoon black pepper

pinch of nutmeg

12 eggs, separated

200g (7oz) feta cheese, crumbled

Preheat the oven to 200°C/400°F/Gas Mark 6.

First, cook the frozen spinach, just for 2 minutes. Once cooled, squeeze it really well, so that all the juices are removed; this is crucial. You can use cheese cloth, but I usually use clean hands and just keep squeezing until the mixture is quite dry. Stir in the pepper and nutmeg and set aside.

Whisk the egg whites until they are firm. Now give the egg yolks a good whisk and crumble in the feta (keep the pieces delicate so you have a good mix throughout). Do not whisk, but give it a little stir. Stir the dry spinach into the egg yolk, then gently fold in the egg whites.

Divide between the 12 holes of a muffin tray or pour into a small baking tray.

Place in the centre of the oven and bake for 10 minutes, taking care not to open the oven. Open the door and allow the soufflés to cool a little in the oven, before allowing them to cool fully at room temperature.

③ Cheddar, Thyme & Caramelized Onion Ⓥ

Makes 12

1 tablespoon olive oil

2 red onions, finely sliced

1 teaspoon dried thyme

1 tablespoon good balsamic vinegar

12 eggs, separated

200g (2 cups) finely grated mature Cheddar

sea salt and black pepper

Preheat the oven to 200°C/400°F/Gas Mark 6.

Pour the oil into a frying pan over a low heat, add the onions and thyme and very slowly cook until they are sticky and caramelized. Increase the heat, add the balsamic and deglaze the pan. Set aside.

Whisk the egg whites until they are firm. Now give the egg yolks a good whisk, crumble in the cheddar and season. Do not whisk, but give it a little stir. Now fold in the egg whites.

Line each muffin hollow or case with the caramelized onion, then pour in the egg mixture. Place in the centre of the oven and bake for 10 minutes, taking care not to open the oven. Open the door and allow the soufflés to cool a little in the oven, before allowing them to cool fully at room temperature.

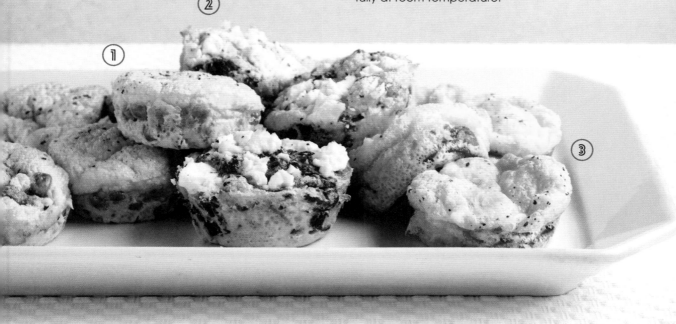

NUT BUTTERS

I simply love nut butters, as they're a quick and totally delicious way to throw together a two-minute snack, ticking off a little bit of fat to keep you full and some protein and fibre from the nuts. I can count the times I have made my own nut butter from scratch on one hand; yes, they're fabulous, but to be honest, I buy whole nut butters with no sugar added and tweak them a little for variety – as in the concoctions here. There are wonderful sugar-free options available and I'm just far too lazy to make from scratch. I make my own little combinations and store them in preserve jars. I prepare these in bulk, using 2–3 jars, but start with a little batch and experiment with your own blends until you find your favourite. These are hardly recipes, but I hope they encourage you to cheat and experiment. Here are some of our family favourites. If you're having these as a snack then 1 portion is 1 tablespoon.

① Chocolate Hazelnut (Vg)

The espresso just brings out the taste of the chocolate, but you can absolutely leave it out. Add some chopped hazelnuts for more texture and adjust the sweetness and chocolate factor to suit you, just make sure you are using pure cocoa powder with no added sugar.

Makes 1 jar

175g (6oz) jar of sugar-free hazelnut butter

2 teaspoons cocoa powder

¼ teaspoon espresso powder

stevia, to taste

All I do is open a little jar, drain off the oil, blend it into some cocoa powder and espresso powder with a pinch of stevia and give it a super-good blend with a spoon. Stir back into the jar of nut butter and you've got a cheat's hazelnut chocolate spread that the whole family will love.

② Cashew, Coconut & Vanilla (Vg)

This makes a great gift that looks like you've made an effort. It ticks off the coconut crush without the hidden sugars found in so many coconut yogurts and is a firm favourite with my girls.

Makes 1 jar

seeds of 1 vanilla pod, or ½ teaspoon vanilla paste

175g (6oz) jar of sugar-free cashew nut butter

1 tablespoon salted roasted cashew nuts, chopped

1 tablespoon desiccated coconut

Simply scrape the vanilla seeds from the pod and stir into the jar of nut butter (or just stir in the vanilla paste), along with the salted roasted cashew nuts and desiccated coconut.

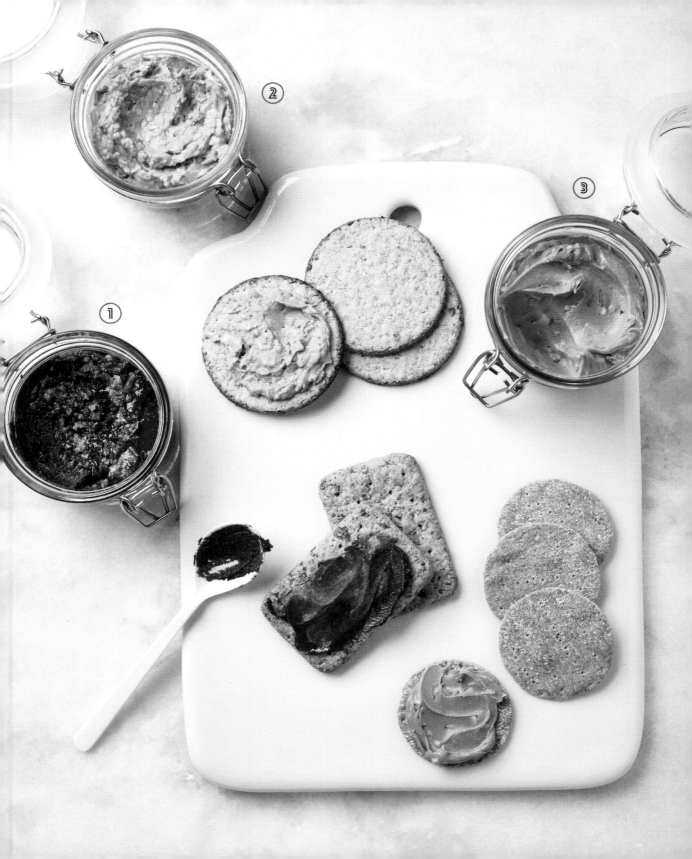

③ Candied Nut Butter Ⓥ

This uses the cinnamon nuts that are a staple snack in Lean for Life. This recipe makes more nuts than you need to make the butter but they make a great snack and will stay fresh in an airtight jar for up to 2 weeks. Again, it's a really quick cheat's recipe that's hardly a recipe at all. But it's a little pot of heaven.

Makes 2 jars

2 x 175g (6oz) jars of smooth peanut butter

3 tablespoons Cinnamon Nuts (see below), chopped finely

FOR THE CINNAMON NUTS

1 egg white

70g (½ cup) almonds

70g (½ cup) cashews

50g (½ cup) pecan nuts

50g (½ cup) walnuts

¾ teaspoon stevia

½ teaspoon sea salt

2 teaspoons ground cinnamon

To make the Cinnamon Nuts, preheat the oven to 160°C/325°F/Gas Mark 3.

Whip the egg white, then fold in the nuts, stevia, half the sea salt and half the cinnamon. Throw on to a lightly oiled baking tray and bake for 15 minutes, stirring every 5 minutes.

Remove from the oven and stir in the rest of the sea salt and cinnamon.

To make the nut butter, finely chop 3 tablespoons of the cinnamon nuts, stir into the peanut butter and store in a preserve jar.

⟵ *illustrated on previous page*

Seedy Strawbs (Vg)

A couple of tablespoons of this and a piece of fruit makes a fast, fit snack.

Makes 1 jar

1 tablespoon olive oil

1 teaspoon sea salt

1 teaspoon red chilli flakes

1 teaspoon sweet paprika

130g (1 cup) pumpkin seeds

150g (1 cup) sesame seeds

2 tablespoons dehydrated strawberries

Preheat the oven to 160°C/325°F/Gas Mark 3.

Stir the olive oil, salt, red chilli and paprika in a bowl until combined, then add the seeds and stir well. Tip the seeds onto a baking tray and bake for 10 minutes, until the pumpkin seeds begin to pop. Remove and allow to cool. Once cool, add the strawberries and store in an airtight jar for up to 2 weeks.

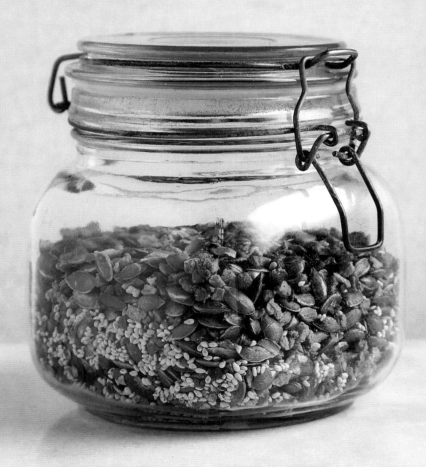

ROASTED SNACKS 4 WAYS

Do interchange the pulses, nuts and seasonings and just use my very basic recipe as a guide. Pouch them up in little zip lock bags so you can grab a pack or two as you're running out the door in the morning. This is a quick weekend job and so worth the effort. Have 2 tablespoons and a low-GI fruit as a snack.

① Chocolate Cinnamon Almonds (Vg)

Each serving is 2 tablespoons

280g (2 cups) almonds, skin on

1 tablespoon cocoa powder

½ teaspoon stevia

½ teaspoon ground cinnamon

Preheat the oven to 160°C/325°F/Gas Mark 3.

Bake the almonds for 10 minutes, giving them a shake halfway through. Turn off the oven.

Place the almonds in a bowl with the cocoa, stevia and cinnamon and stir to coat well. Return to the baking tray and leave to cool in the oven, with the door slightly ajar.

Cool completely, then store in an airtight jar for up to 2 weeks.

② Ras El Hanout Roasted Chickpeas (Vg)

Each serving is 2 tablespoons

2 x 400g (14oz) cans chickpeas, drained and rinsed

1 tablespoon ras el hanout

sea salt and black pepper

2 tablespoons groundnut oil

1 tablespoons rose petals (obviously not vital)

Preheat the oven to 180°C/350°F/Gas Mark 4.

Dry the chickpeas on a kitchen towel. Mix together the ras el hanout, salt and pepper and oil in a bowl and toss in the chickpeas to coat. Lie them flat on a baking tray and simply bake for 30 minutes until they are dry and crispy. Every 10 minutes, give the pan a little shake.

Once they are cooled, sprinkle them with the rose petals; these are purely for decoration so really don't lose any sleep over not finding them! Cool completely, then store in an airtight jar for up to 5 days if using rose petals, 2 weeks if not.

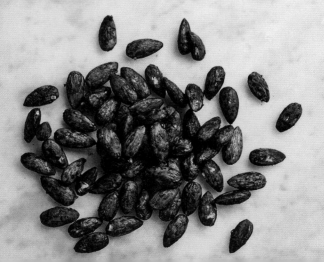

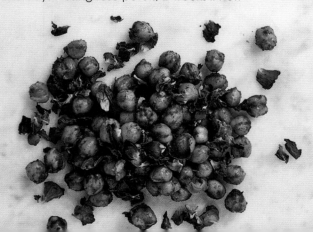

③ Winter Nuts ⓥ

Each serving is 2 tablespoons

1 egg white

70g (½ cup) almonds

65g (½ cup) cashews

50g (½ cup) pecan nuts

50g (½ cup) walnuts

½–1 teaspoon stevia, to taste

½ teaspoon sea salt

½ teaspoon ground allspice

½ teaspoon ground cinnamon

½ teaspoon freshly grated nutmeg

½ teaspoon finely grated unwaxed orange zest

a little olive oil

Preheat the oven to 160°C/325°F/Gas Mark 3.

Whisk the egg white, then fold in all the nuts with the stevia, half the sea salt, allspice, cinnamon, nutmeg and orange zest.

Throw on to a lightly oiled baking tray and bake for 15 minutes, stirring the nuts every 5 minutes.

Remove from the oven and stir in the remainder of the seasonings. Cool completely, then store in an airtight jar for up to 2 weeks.

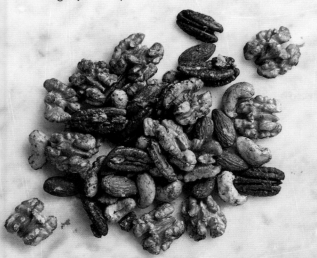

④ Sweet Lanka Nuts ⓥ

Each serving is 2 tablespoons

1 egg white

130g (1 cup) cashews

65g (½ cup) shelled pistachio nuts

70g (½ cup) almonds, skin on

½–1 teaspoon stevia, to taste

½ teaspoon sea salt

½ teaspoon black pepper

½ teaspoon garam masala

½ teaspoon ground cinnamon

a little olive oil

1 teaspoon cumin seeds

1 teaspoon fennel seeds

Preheat the oven to 160°C/325°F/Gas Mark 3.

Whisk the egg white, then fold in all the nuts with the stevia, half the sea salt, black pepper, garam masala and cinnamon.

Throw on to a lightly oiled baking tray and bake for 15 minutes, stirring the nuts every 5 minutes. After 5 minutes, add all the cumin and fennel seeds.

Remove from the oven and stir in the remainder of the seasonings. Cool completely, then store in an airtight jar for up to 2 weeks.

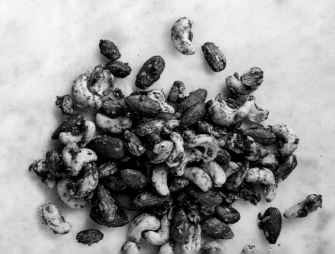

Double Deckers (Vg)

These are a bit messy for work and travel, but great for at home days with a comforting cup of tea. They make for a great snack on higher energy days.

Serves 2

12 mini oatcakes

6 tablespoons chocolate hazelnut butter (see page 60)

1 banana, sliced

To make each double decker, take 3 mini oatcakes, layering 1½ tablespoons of the chocolate hazelnut butter and a slice of banana between each layer (works wonderfully with slices of strawberry too, if you fancy a lower-carb option).

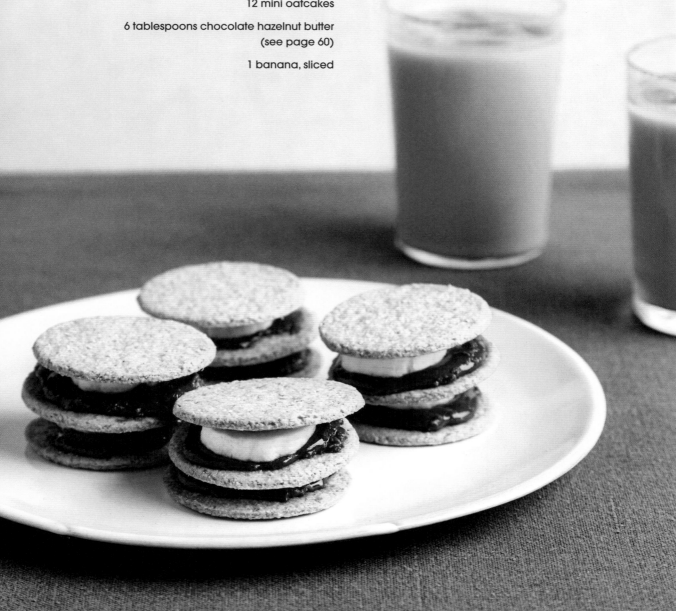

HUMMUS 3 WAYS

Any of these make a great weekend snack and you can vary the flavourings in so many ways. Add a tablespoon of good harissa or smoked chilli paste, green or red pesto, 8 large green or black olives or a handful of spinach, basil, kale or parsley for an extra taste sensation. You can use shop-bought cooked peppers, or try it with artichoke too. Experiment! Obviously it's not essential to skin the chickpeas, but it does make for a really creamy hummus. If you like a looser consistency, simply add more lime or lemon. Your portion of hummus here is 2 tablespoons and serve it with wholemeal pitta chips (see below) or crudités.

① My Basic Hummus (Vg)

Each serving is 2 tablespoons

FOR THE PITTA CHIPS

2 large wholemeal pitta breads,
cut into eighths

good spray of olive oil

sea salt and black pepper

FOR THE HUMMUS

juice of 1 lemon

2 tablespoons tahini

½ garlic clove (optional)

2 x 400g (14oz) cans chickpeas,
skinned if you have time

sea salt and black pepper

Preheat the oven to 200°C/400°F/Gas Mark 6.

Start with the pitta chips. Spray the pitta pieces with a good dose of oil. Season and bake on a baking tray for 8 minutes until brown and crispy.

Put the lemon juice and seasoning in a food processor with the tahini and garlic and blend for 30 seconds. Now add the chickpeas and blend until super-smooth.

② Roast Pepper (Vg)

Each serving is 2 tablespoons

1 Romano pepper

juice of ½ lime, plus pinch unwaxed lime zest

4 tablespoons tahini

½ garlic clove

2 x 400g (14oz) cans chickpeas,
skinned if you have time

½ teaspoon chilli flakes

sea salt and black pepper

Preheat the oven to 240°C/475°F/Gas Mark 9.

Place the pepper, whole, on a baking tray in the middle of the oven. I don't bother to deseed or oil it, just give it a quick rinse under the tap. Bake for 20–25 minutes until soft and caramelized. Once cooled a little, cut the stalk ends off and, over the sink, squeeze out the pips and liquid. Now roughly chop the flesh.

In a food processor, add the lime juice, seasoning, pepper, tahini and garlic and blend together for 30 seconds. Add the chickpeas and blend until super-smooth. Add the chilli flakes and pulse for 15 seconds. Finally, stir in the zest and season to taste.

③ El Verde (Vg)

Each serving is 2 tablespoons

juice of 1 lime

1 ripe avocado

½ mild green chilli, deseeded

½ garlic clove

400g (14oz) can chickpeas,
skinned if you have time

400g (14oz) can cannellini beans

small handful of coriander, chopped

sea salt and black pepper

In a food processor, add the lime juice, seasoning, avocado, chilli and garlic and blend for 30 seconds. Now add the chickpeas and beans and blend until super-smooth. Finally add the coriander – as much as you wish – and pulse just for 15 seconds.

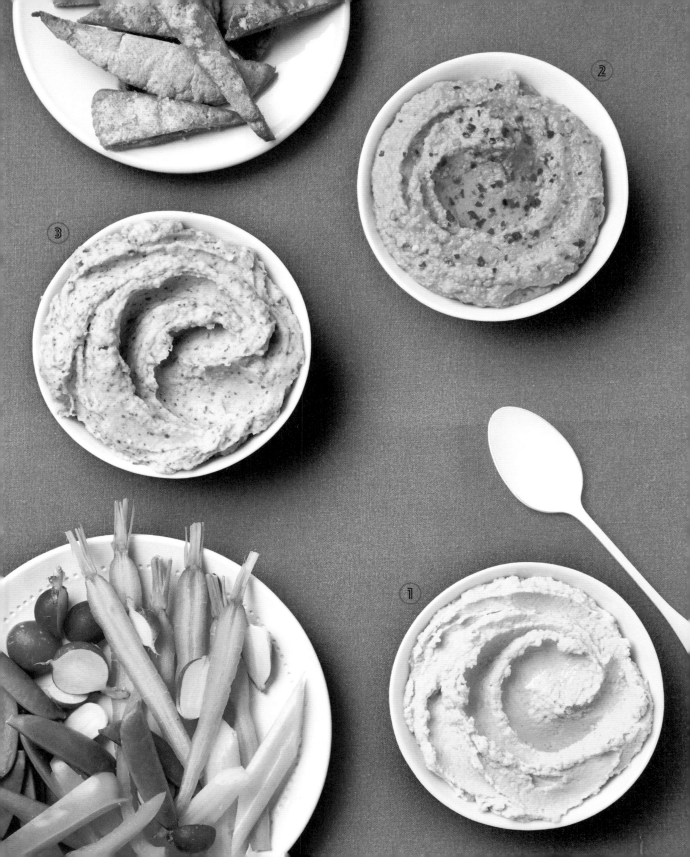

DIPS 3 WAYS

These dips and whips can be adapted to your heart's content. Play around, always add protein and eat with wholemeal crackers and crudités. These make a great weekend snack, but you can pot them up and take into work too. The more prepared you are to prepare ahead, the more variety you're going to have in your new lifestyle. Give it a go. Each serving is 2 tablespoons.

① Spiced Cream Cheese ⓥ

Each serving is 2 tablespoons

200g (¾ cup) quark

200g (¾ cup) ricotta cheese

1 teaspoon vanilla paste

½ teaspoon finely grated unwaxed orange zest

½ teaspoon finely grated unwaxed lemon zest

pinch of freshly grated nutmeg

pinch of ground cinnamon

½ teaspoon stevia

Combine the quark, ricotta and vanilla in a bowl, and mix well using a wooden spoon. Add the remaining ingredients bit by bit, until you are happy with the flavour.

② Chocolate & Walnut Whip ⓥ

Each serving is 2 tablespoons

100g (1 cup) walnuts

200g (¾ cup) low-fat cream cheese

100g (⅓ cup) Greek yogurt

1½ teaspoons cocoa powder

½ teaspoon vanilla paste

½ teaspoon stevia

Firstly, toast the walnuts in a dry wok, taking care not to brown them too much. Set aside to cool.

In a food processor, blend together the cream cheese, Greek yogurt, cocoa powder and vanilla paste until it is nicely whipped. Add in the stevia, to taste and blend for a further 15 seconds.

Only when the walnuts are totally cool (I put mine in the freezer for 10 minutes), add to the mix and pulse for 5–10 seconds, just until they are blended through, but still a bit chunky.

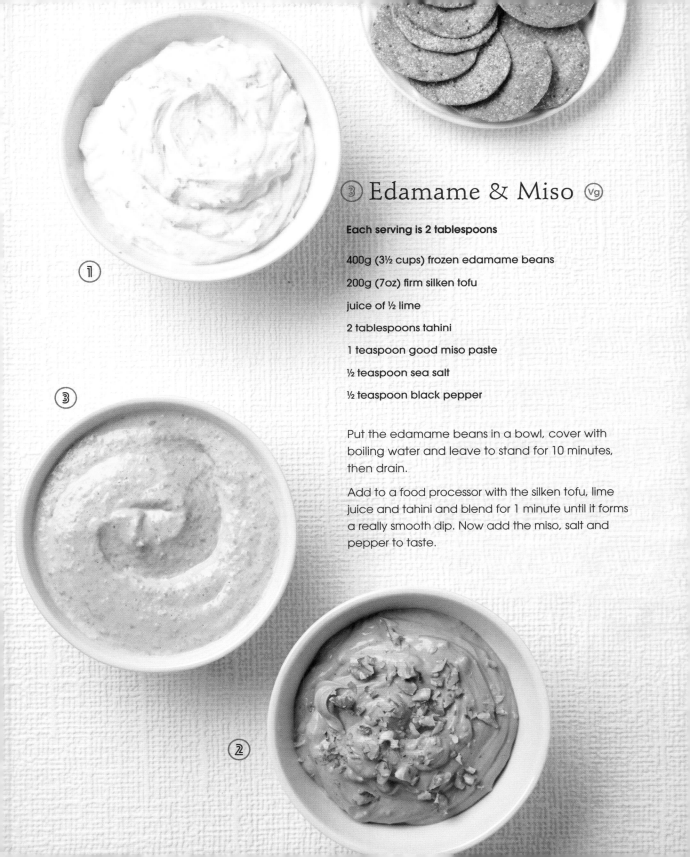

③ Edamame & Miso (Vg)

Each serving is 2 tablespoons

400g (3½ cups) frozen edamame beans

200g (7oz) firm silken tofu

juice of ½ lime

2 tablespoons tahini

1 teaspoon good miso paste

½ teaspoon sea salt

½ teaspoon black pepper

Put the edamame beans in a bowl, cover with boiling water and leave to stand for 10 minutes, then drain.

Add to a food processor with the silken tofu, lime juice and tahini and blend for 1 minute until it forms a really smooth dip. Now add the miso, salt and pepper to taste.

HOW TO BUILD A SMOOTHIE OR SMOOTHIE BOWL

These smoothies are really intended as a snack, but you can increase the quantities, or add a handful of nuts, if you want to use them as a little meal substitute on a night when you get home late and don't feel very hungry. Another option is to increase the amount of protein and oatbran by 50 per cent and turn your smoothie into a smoothie bowl.

My favourite base is Greek yogurt, as it's strained of water and so has super protein powers. The mild flavour forms a great base for smoothies or smoothie bowls.

Any of these smoothies can be turned into smoothie bowls, by simply reducing the liquid in the recipe and adding extra oatbran. Smoothies are fantastic for drinking on the go, or for a hurried breakfast when you're putting your make-up on, but it's sometimes just good to sit down and eat your smoothie with a spoon... It also involves the kids in healthy eating by giving them a great canvas for decorating to their hearts' content.

Many of you have asked for vegan versions, and so I've included a good handful here with a base of soya yogurt or silken tofu. Any recipe with 100g (3½oz) of Greek yogurt will require just over twice that amount of soya yogurt or silken tofu to roughly get the same amount of protein, which would give you more smoothie than you want. It's not a deal breaker if you have a smoothie with a lower level of protein; the main thing is that you always have a dose of protein in every meal or snack. You can increase the amount of soya yogurt or silken tofu in any smoothie if you want more protein, but be aware that you'll need to adjust the consistency by adding more water, as it will be thick. Please feel free to experiment and use the following pages to come up with your own flavour concoctions.

Alternatively, you can use a protein powder. Protein powders are a fantastic, easy source of protein and I'd recommend a whey, pea or soy protein powder; just ensure that each scoop contains roughly 20g (½oz) of protein and is low in sugars, and you're set. Keep an eye on the carbs: aim for a powder with the lowest carbs that you can find, so we can add carbs in a more delicious form instead, such as fresh or frozen fruit.

Do keep the freezer stacked with a variety of frozen fruit; it really is abundantly full of vitamins as it is flash-frozen at the time of picking and doesn't sit in storage containers for weeks. Plus, it is ready washed, peeled and available 365 days a year.

You'll see I use oatbran in most of these smoothie recipes; I really think it's the most precious ingredient. It's abundantly high in fibre, will keep you full for longer and – ensuring it's blended well – add some thickness to your smoothie or smoothie bowl. Oatbran is proven to reduce bad cholesterol and I try to have at least a tablespoon or two a day.

Smoothies do tend to be as good as the blender you are using. Powerful, professional blenders are damn expensive, but they do give such a creamy and more intensely flavoured hit to smoothies and soups. Keep your eye out for second-hand options, they're so worth the investment. I've had my Vitamix for more than five years and use it at least a couple of times a day.

→ *smoothie toppings illustrated overleaf*

WHERE'S THE PROTEIN?

This should always be your first question with any LP Method meal or snack.
Protein is essential to stablize your blood sugars and, crucially, to maintain muscle as you drop body fat.

Greek yoghurt ★ protein powder (whey, pea, vegan) ★ tofu ★ soy yoghurt

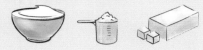

ADD A FIBRE FREEBIE

I add oat bran to every smoothie that I make. It's 50 per cent higher in fibre than normal oats (helping to stabilize blood sugar levels), keeps you fuller for longer, is great for bowel health and reduces cholesterol.

oat bran

DO I NEED A SEPARATE HEALTHY FAT?

Dietary 'healthy' fats are essential to help the body burn fat as efficiently as possible. If you use low-fat yoghurt, add in a separate fat like a few nuts, seeds, a dash of omega oils or nut butter for extra taste and texture. If not, use a fuller fat yoghurt.

seeds ★ nuts ★ oil blends (such as Udo's oils) ★ nut butters

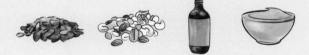

LOVE LOWER-GI CARB FLAVOURS

Lower-GI carbs will give you the energy you need to fuel your day whilst still allowing you to burn through fat storage. They're also a great source of flavour and antioxidants.

frozen fruits ★ fresh fruits

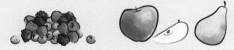

SMOOTHIE OR SMOOTHIE BOWL?

Smoothie bowls make a lovely change from a smoothie, letting you play around with extra goodies on top too. Simply add more oatbran and less liquid for a thicker consistency.

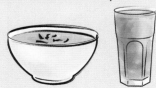

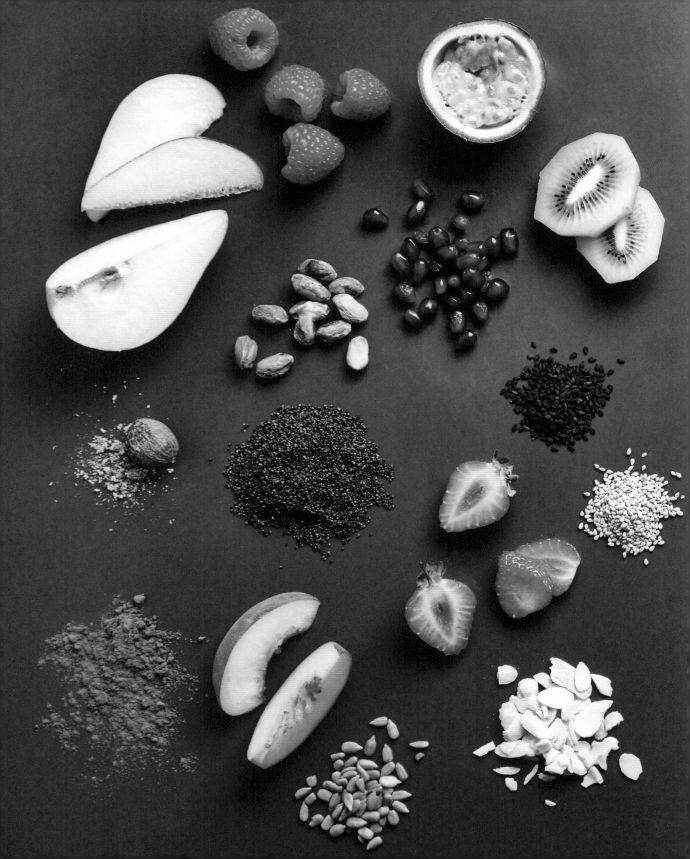

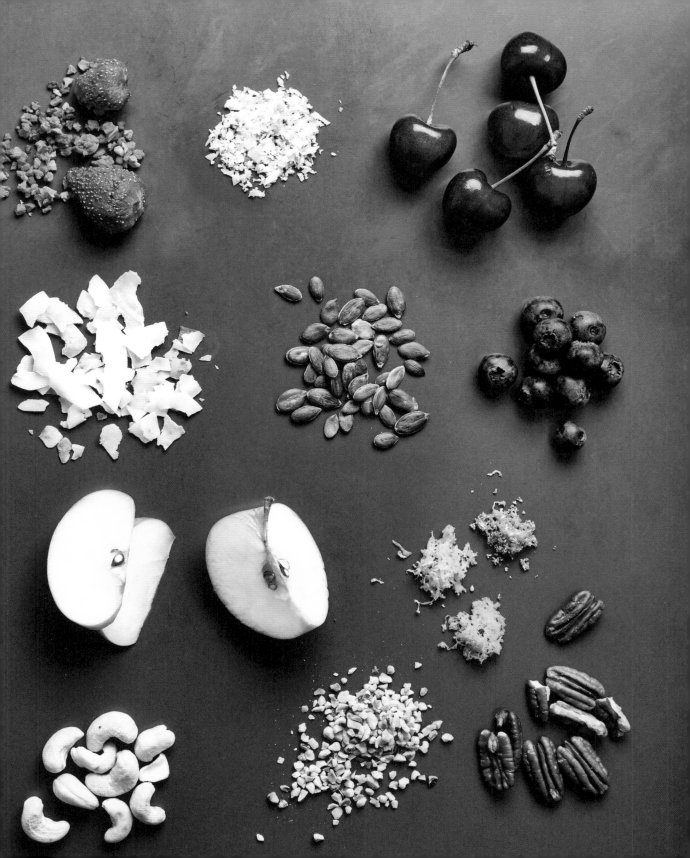

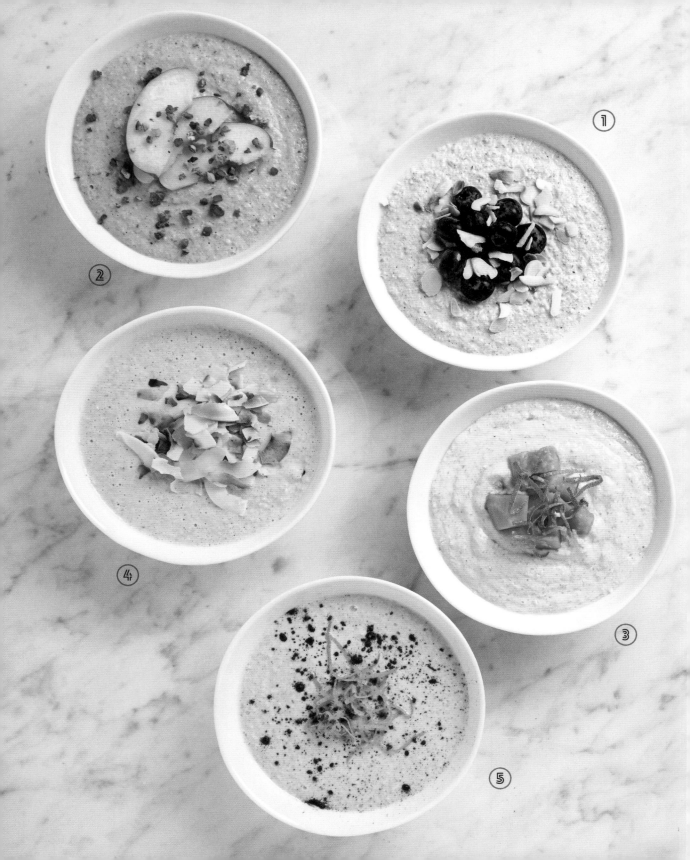

5 SMOOTHIE BOWLS

These are really just versions of my protein smoothies that are thicker, so you should be able to eat with a spoon. They just make a lovely change and I throw little pots of toppings on the table for everyone to help themselves. Adjust the consistency to what suits you and don't be a slave to the recipes. Ideally use a very powerful blender to make these, then simply add more ice, water or milk to change into a drinkable smoothie.

① Vanilla & Almond ⓥ

Serves 1

100g (⅓ cup) low-fat Greek yogurt

½ teaspoon vanilla paste

1 tablespoon almond butter

1 tablespoon oatbran

100ml milk (scant ½ cup), or to taste

pinch of stevia, to taste

FOR THE TOPPINGS (OPTIONAL)

toasted flaked almonds

blueberries

Blend all the ingredients except the stevia together for 1 minute until smooth. Adjust the amount of milk to achieve your desired consistency, then taste and sweeten with stevia to taste.

Serve the smoothie in a bowl with the almonds and blueberries, or choose your own toppings.

② Peach & Strawbs ⓥ

Serves 1

1 peach, skin on, halved and stoned

20 strawberries

100g (⅓ cup) Greek yogurt

1 tablespoon oatbran

½ teaspoon vanilla paste

milk or water, to taste

stevia, to taste

FOR THE TOPPINGS (OPTIONAL)

dried strawberries

fresh sliced peaches

Preheat the oven to 200°C/400°F/Gas Mark 6.

Place the peach halves and strawberries on a baking tray and bake for 15 minutes, then allow to cool. Blend with the yogurt, oatbran and vanilla for 1 minute.

Add enough milk or water to achieve your desired consistency, then taste and add stevia to taste.

Serve the smoothie in a bowl with the dried strawberries and fresh sliced peaches, or choose your own toppings.

③ Mango, Papaya & Lime ⓥ

Serves 1

100g (⅓ cup) Greek yogurt

50g (1¾oz) papaya, fresh or frozen

50g (1¾oz) mango, frozen

pinch of finely grated unwaxed lime zest

1 tablespoon oatbran

FOR THE TOPPINGS (OPTIONAL)

unwaxed lime zest, finely grated

papaya, coarsely chopped

Blend all the ingredients for 1 minute until super-smooth. Serve the smoothie in a bowl with the lime zest and papaya, or choose your own toppings.

④ Coconut, Vanilla & Cashew ⓥ

Serves 1

100g (⅓ cup) Greek yogurt

1 tablespoon oatbran

1 tablespoon cashew nut butter

1 tablespoon unsweetened desiccated coconut

stevia, to taste

½ teaspoon vanilla paste

dash of milk, or coconut water, to taste

FOR THE TOPPING (OPTIONAL)

toasted coconut flakes

Blend all the ingredients except the milk or coconut water for 1 minute until super-smooth. Add milk or coconut water to achieve your desired consistency. Serve the smoothie in a bowl with the coconut flakes, or choose your own toppings.

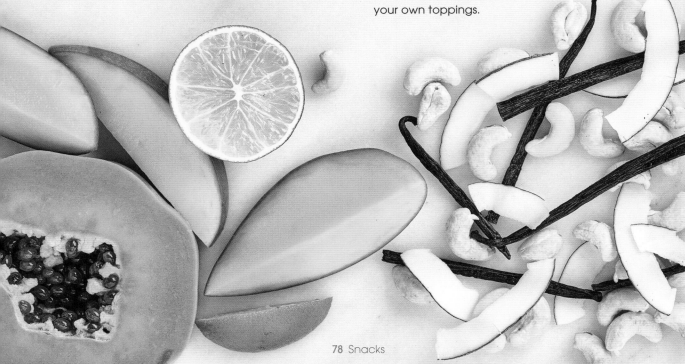

⑤ Baked Pear, Apple & Cinnamon Ⓥ

Serves 1

½ pear, skin on, halved and cored

½ apple, skin on, halved and cored

100g (⅓ cup) Greek yogurt

1 tablespoon oatbran

½ teaspoon vanilla paste

½ teaspoon ground cinnamon

milk or water, to taste

FOR THE TOPPINGS (OPTIONAL)

dusting of ground cinnamon

unwaxed orange zest, finely grated

Preheat the oven to 200°C/400°F/Gas Mark 6.

Bake the pear and apple for 15 minutes, then allow to cool.

Blend the apple and pear with the yogurt, oatbran, vanilla and cinnamon for 1 minute until super-smooth. Stir in enough milk or water to achieve your desired consistency. Serve the smoothie in a bowl with the cinnamon and orange zest, or choose your own toppings.

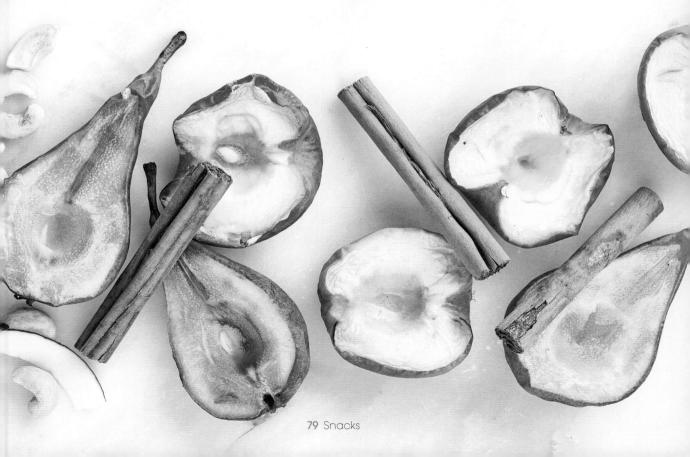

5 SMOOTHIES

My Vitality Smoothie in *Lean for Life* is something I probably have 200 days a year. I just swear by the powers of the frozen fruits. But here are some more smoothie options, including a vegan Vitality version. It would need up to 250g (1 cup) soya yogurt to get a similar protein quota as the Greek yogurt version but, consistency wise, the recipe works better with 200g (¾ cup). Again, play around with a consistency that suits you and experiment with other low-GI fruits and flavours. Keep ringing the changes.

① Strawberry Sour ⓥ

Serves 1

200g (¾ cup) soya yogurt, or silken tofu, or 1 scoop of vegan protein powder

100g (¾ cup) ripe or frozen strawberries

½ red grapefruit

1 tablespoon oatbran

stevia, to taste

Blend all the ingredients except the stevia together for 1 minute until smooth. Adjust the amount of water to achieve your desired consistency, then taste and sweeten with stevia to taste.

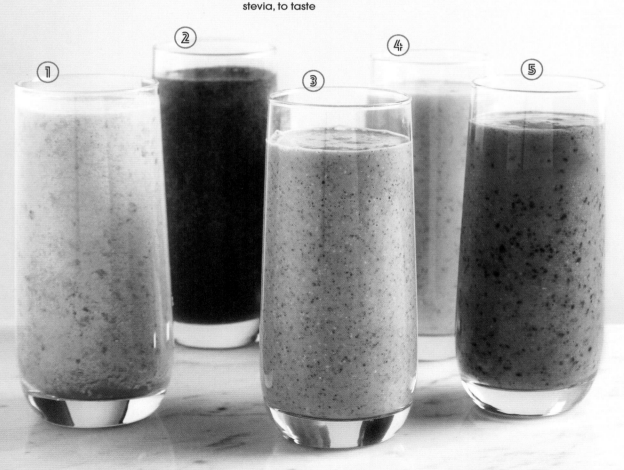

② Chocolate Cherry Ⓥ

Serves 1

1 scoop of chocolate protein powder

100g (¾ cup) frozen cherries

1 teaspoon cocoa powder

1 tablespoon oatbran

semi-skimmed (1 or 2%) milk,
or unsweetened soya milk, to taste

stevia, to taste

Blend all the ingredients except the milk and
stevia together for 1 minute until smooth. Adjust
the amount of milk to achieve your desired
consistency, then taste and sweeten with stevia
to taste.

④ Blood Orange Ⓥg

Serves 1

1 scoop of vanilla protein powder

100g (¾ cup) frozen raspberries

1 blood orange, peeled

1 tablespoon oatbran

½ teaspoon vanilla paste

soya milk, to taste

stevia, to taste

Blend all the ingredients except the milk and
stevia together for 1 minute until smooth. Adjust
the amount of milk to achieve your desired
consistency, then taste and sweeten with stevia
to taste.

③ Apple & Greens Ⓥg

Serves 1

200g (¾ cup) soya yogurt, or silken tofu,
or 1 scoop of vegan protein powder

1 green apple, cored, skin on

½ cucumber

4–6 mint sprigs

small handful of flat leaf parsley

small handful of spinach

1 teaspoon oatbran

Ice cubes, to taste

Blend all the ingredients together for 90 seconds
until smooth. Add water if necessary to achieve
your desired consistency.

⑤ Vegan Vitality Ⓥg

Serves 1

200g (¾ cup) soya yogurt, or silken tofu,
or 1 scoop of vegan protein powder

100g (¾ cup) frozen summer berries

50g (¼ cup) blueberries

1 tablespoon oatbran

stevia, to taste

Blend all the ingredients except the stevia
together for 1 minute until smooth. Adjust the
amount of water to achieve your desired
consistency, then taste and sweeten with stevia
to taste.

3
SOUPS

There's nothing quite as comforting as a hot bowl of fresh soup. It provides a little smug factor, too, that you've made something from scratch, often out of the contents of the fridge drawer, that is so warming and comforting – like a hug in a bowl. And soups are so ridiculously simple to make, once you get the principle, and provide abundantly more vitamins and minerals than any shop-bought variety… not to mention so much more flavour. They're the best way of using up leftovers too, and the less food we waste, the better. There are endless varieties and here I include some of my family favourites, but do tweak them and experiment. Just don't forget the protein. Whether it's a snack or main meal, always ask yourself: 'Where is the protein?'. It's the key to regulating your appetite and maintaining your muscle mass and metabolism as you lose body fat.

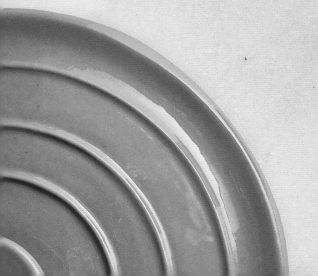

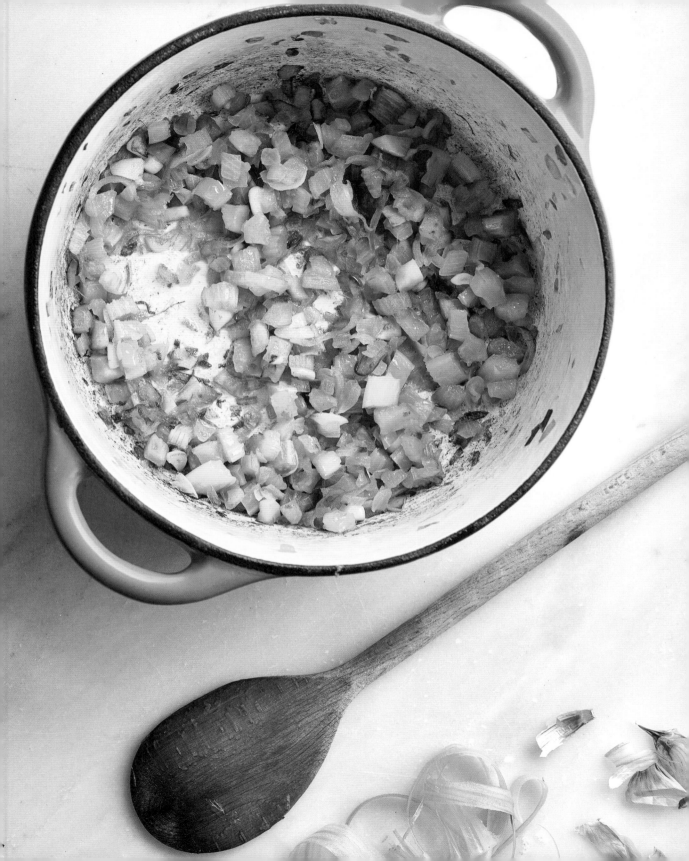

HOW TO BUILD A SOUP

WHERE'S THE PROTEIN?

Often you'll find you prepare the protein separately, adding it to the soup already cooked.

meat ★ fish ★ soya proteins ★ beans & pulses

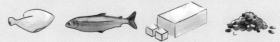

START BY SAUTÉING THE BASE

Every soup needs a good base to build upon. Sauté these ingredients gently in a little oil until softened. Be careful not to cook too quickly and burn them.

celery ★ onion ★ carrot

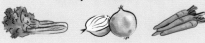

STOCK UP ON FLAVOUR

After the base, add the stock. Your stock contributes a lot of the deep flavours in your soup and so if you make your own with cooking juices then you'll see a big difference. If there's no time to make your own stock then the ready-made options available now are a brilliant cheat.

stock ★ wine (just a dash) ★ miso

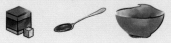

LOW-GI VEG

Add extra veggies to your soup – either fresh or frozen. Don't overcook them as you want a little bite. When cooked, keep the soup chunky or blend for a smoother texture.

peas ★ sweetcorn ★ carrots ★ broccoli ★ cauliflower ★ mushrooms ★ tomatoes ★ red peppers ★ green beans

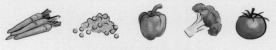

A LITTLE SPRINKLE

It can be tempting to overlook the last finishing touches but they really do make a difference. Whether it's to add a crunch, a little extra zing or some extra richness, take time to try new toppings.

toasted nuts ★ fresh herbs & chillies ★ cream (just a dash) ★ grated cheese ★ citrus juices

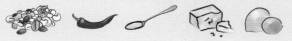

Aduki & Flageolet Bean

Serves 4

400g (14oz) can flageolet beans, drained and rinsed

400g (14oz) can aduki beans, drained and rinsed

1–1.5 litres (4–6 cups) good chicken or vegetable stock

2 garlic cloves, finely sliced

1 tablespoon olive oil

1 onion, finely chopped

1 celery stick, finely chopped

1 carrot, finely chopped

8 ripe tomatoes, chopped

1 teaspoon good pesto

leaves from 1 bunch of basil

sea salt and black pepper

100g (1 cup) Parmesan cheese, finely grated

good handful of flat leaf parsley leaves, chopped

Aduki beans are a fabulous source of protein and packed with vitamins – but use any beans that you have lurking in the cupboard. I always use canned but you can soak your own of course, I just can't be bothered. As long as you've got some basic veggies available, you can prepare this comforting meal in minutes.

Tip the beans into a casserole dish with 1 litre (4 cups) of the stock and the garlic. Bring to the boil, then reduce the heat to low and simmer for 15 minutes.

Meanwhile, heat the olive oil in a large non-stick frying pan and add the onion, celery and carrot. Sauté for 6 minutes over a medium heat until soft. Add the tomatoes and continue cooking for another 4 minutes.

Now simply mix the vegetables into the pan of beans and stock, add the pesto and basil and simmer gently for a couple of minutes just until the flavours combine. Taste and add up to another 500ml (2 cups) of water or stock if needed and check for seasoning, adjusting to taste.

Serve in bowls with the grated Parmesan and parsley sprinkled over.

→ *illustrated overleaf, bottom bowl*

Miso, Ginger & Edamame ⓥ

Serves 4

1½ tablespoons groundnut oil

200g (2⅔ cups) shiitake mushrooms, chopped

4 spring onions, finely sliced lengthways, white parts only

2 carrots, halved, finely sliced lengthways

1 yellow pepper, finely chopped

400g (14oz) firm tofu, cubed

1 tablespoon good-quality miso paste

1–1.5 litres (4–6 cups) hot water

120g (1 cup) frozen edamame beans

a little fresh root ginger, peeled and finely chopped

200g (about 1 head) pak choi, finely sliced

200g (2 cups) beansprouts

1 teaspoon sesame oil

1 tablespoon reduced-sodium soy sauce, or to taste

black sesame seeds, to serve

leaves from 1 bunch of coriander or flat leaf parsley, finely chopped

Don't be deterred by the ingredient list: this is a quickie to make and when you've cooked it once, you'll be in the groove and your cupboards stocked. It's much simpler than it looks.

Heat 1 tablespoon of the groundnut oil in a non-stick saucepan over a medium heat. Add the mushrooms and white bits of the spring onions and fry until the mushrooms are nearly dry. Now add the carrots and yellow pepper and sauté for 4 minutes. Remove from the pan and set aside.

Blot the tofu dry with kitchen paper. Heat the remaining ½ tablespoon of oil in the pan and brown the tofu gently, turning to colour it on all sides.

Mix the miso paste into 1 litre (4 cups) of the hot water, then pour it into the pan. Throw in the edamame beans and simmer for a minute before adding the ginger, pak choi, beansprouts and sesame oil, as well as the mushroom mixture. Taste, adding the soy sauce if needed and the remaining water if you prefer a milder taste.

Serve sprinkled with the sesame seeds and herbs.

⟶ *illustrated opposite, top bowl*

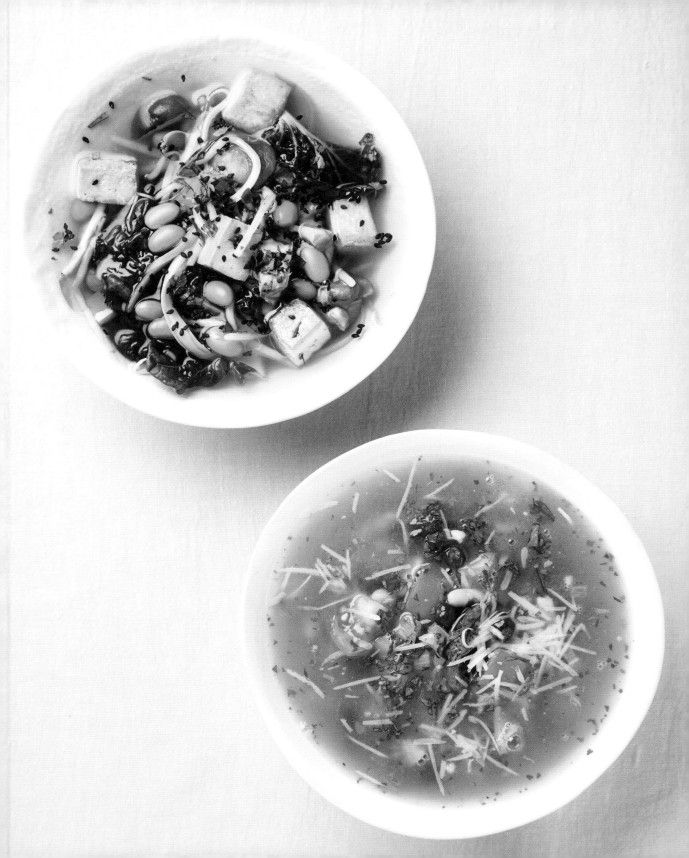

My Tom Yum

Serves 4

4 lemon grass sticks, to taste
(use 2 for your first go)

1–1.5 litres (4–6 cups) water

100g (2 cups) galangal,
peeled and sliced (optional)

6 kaffir lime leaves

12 red tomatoes, quartered

1 red pepper, chopped

2 red chillies, chopped

200g (2⅔ cups) oyster mushrooms, sliced

600g (1lb 5 oz) raw, jumbo king prawns

1 tablespoon fish sauce, to taste

pinch of stevia, to taste

pinch of black pepper

juice of 2 limes, plus lime wedges to serve

leaves from 1 bunch of coriander, chopped

leaves from 1 bunch of Thai basil

1 green tiger chilli, chopped
(optional – tiger chilli is very hot)

Undoubtedly, this is more delicious when you make the paste from scratch, but I often use a good shop-bought paste when I'm in a hurry. It works wonderfully well with chicken and tofu – or a combination of the two. Adjust the stevia and fish sauce to taste, I'm quite heavy handed on flavour here as I really love it to hit all the senses.

Begin by bashing the hell out of the lemon grass; I use a steak tenderizer and give each stick about 10 whacks.

Bring 1 litre (4 cups) of the water to the boil in a saucepan and add the lemon grass, galangal (if using), lime leaves, tomatoes, red pepper, red chillies and mushrooms. Reduce the heat to a gentle simmer and cook for 10 minutes.

Now add the prawns and simmer until they turn pink, about 3–5 minutes, depending on their size. Take the pan off the heat and let it cool a little before tasting. I love my tom yum very rich in flavour, but adjust with the remaining boiling water now if you like.

Add the fish sauce and stevia bit by bit, and some black pepper to adjust the taste. Do this with caution and slowly… too much of either and it's doomed. Now add the lime juice – again, bit by bit – so that you achieve your preferred flavour. Serve up and garnish; I put little bowls of coriander, Thai basil, lime wedges and green tiger chilli out for everyone to help themselves.

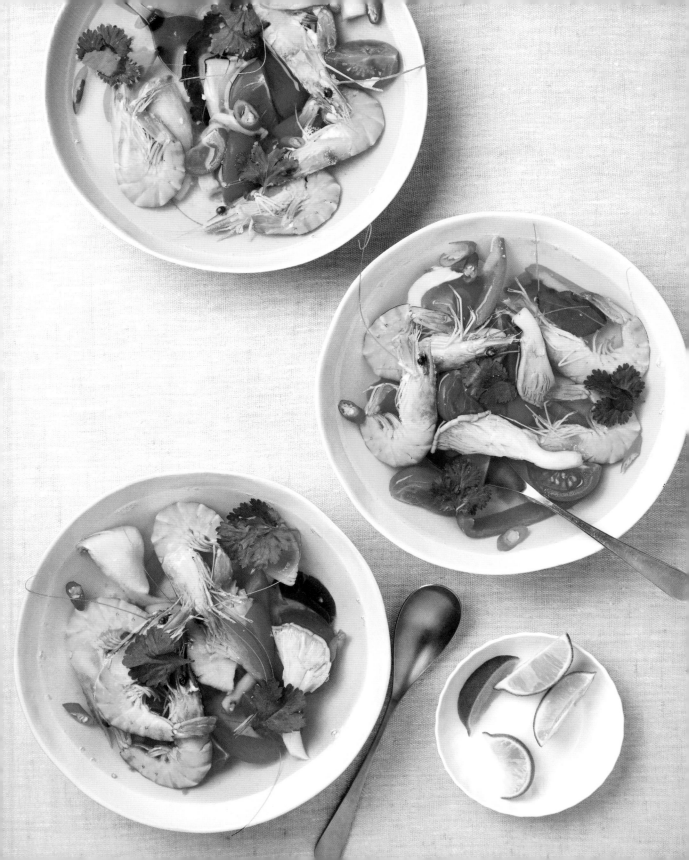

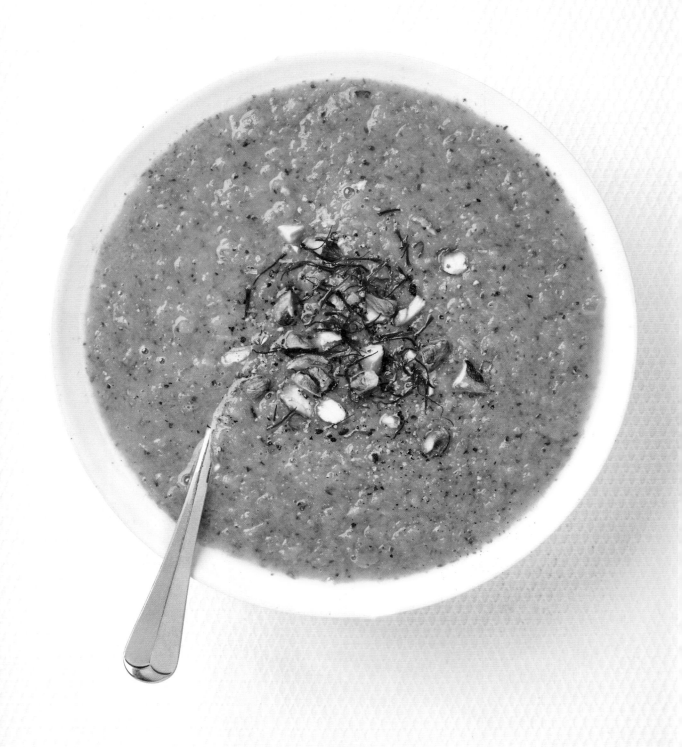

Broccoli, Butter Bean & Pistachio

Serves 4

2 tablespoons olive oil

4 leeks, finely chopped

1 celery stick, finely chopped

1–1.5 litres (4–6 cups) good chicken or vegetable stock

1 head of broccoli, roughly chopped

400g (14oz) can butter beans (preferably skins removed for a smoother soup)

pinch of saffron threads (optional), plus more to serve

50g (scant ½ cup) pistachio nuts, skin off, plus more to serve

sea salt and black pepper

I adore this. It does depend on good stock – but I don't always make my own. This also works wonderfully with leftover shredded chicken or tofu cubes, pan-fried until golden.

In a saucepan, heat the olive oil over a medium heat and gently sauté the leeks and celery until they are translucent. Now add 1 litre (4 cups) of the stock and immerse the broccoli in it.

Add the butter beans and a few threads of saffron and simmer with the lid on until the broccoli is just cooked (about 10 minutes).

Meanwhile, toast the pistachios very gently in a dry pan for 2 minutes over a medium heat to intensify the flavour but not to brown them. Add them to the soup. Taste and season generously.

Transfer, in batches, to a high-speed blender and give it a really good whizz until it is extra smooth. Taste and check whether the consistency and strength is right for you; if not, adjust with the remaining stock.

Pour into bowls and sprinkle with a few more pistachios, chopped, and threads of saffron.

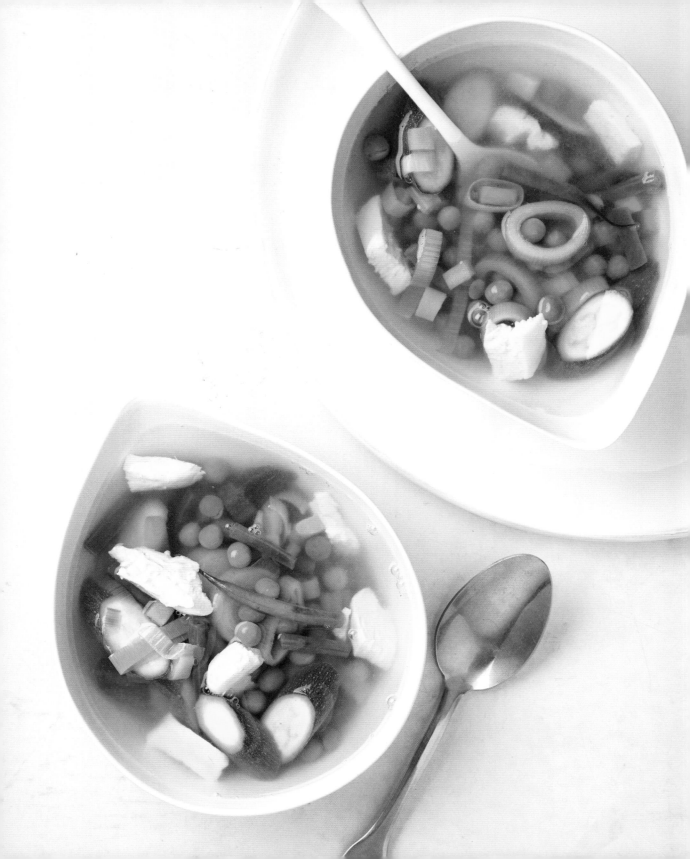

Spring Chicken

Serves 4

600g (1lb 5oz) skinless boneless chicken thigh or breast, or leftover cooked chicken

1–1.5 litres (4–6 cups) good chicken stock

1 tablespoon good olive oil

2 leeks, finely sliced

1 celery stick, finely chopped

2 carrots, finely chopped

1 teaspoon dried herbes de Provençe

1 tablespoon of white wine

200g (1½ cups) green beans, chopped

200g (1½ cups) baby courgettes, chopped

100g (1½ cups) frozen peas

sea salt and black pepper

4 teaspoons good-quality pesto

This is a wonderfully clean and lean soup that I often make on Mondays following the Sunday roast. If I don't have leftovers, I use thighs as they're fuller in flavour. Again, swap in tofu, edamame or beans if you would like a veggie option.

If you're using raw chicken, poach it in the chicken stock for 10–15 minutes (depending on the size) until cooked through, but still tender. Set aside, reserving the stock.

Heat the oil in a saucepan over a medium heat and sauté the leeks, celery, carrots and herbes de Provençe until the leeks are transparent. Pour in the wine and deglaze the pan by stirring to remove all the good brown bits from the base.

Pour in 1 litre (4 cups) of the chicken stock. Bring to the boil, then reduce the heat to a simmer for a couple of minutes. Add the green beans, baby courgettes, peas and chicken, in chunks or chopped, as you prefer, and simmer until all the flavours combine, just for a few minutes, so that the veggies are cooked but still have a little bite to them.

Taste for seasoning, and add more stock if you'd like it thinner. Serve in bowls with a little pesto in each, or if you prefer, a heaped teaspoon each of Parmesan cheese and chopped flat leaf parsley leaves.

Stikini

Serves 4

FOR THE MEATBALLS

2 tablespoons olive oil

1 shallot, finely chopped

1 teaspoon dried herbes de Provençe

100g (1⅓ cups) chanterelles, or other wild mushrooms, finely chopped

1 tablespoon Marsala wine (optional)

1 garlic clove, crushed

300g (1½ cups) minced turkey

300g (1½ cups) minced pork

small handful of flat leaf parsley leaves, chopped

sea salt and black pepper

FOR THE SOUP

2 onions, finely chopped

1 celery stick, finely chopped

½ carrot, finely chopped

100g (½ cup) cherry tomatoes, chopped

1-1.5 litres (4-6 cups) good chicken stock, plus more if needed

pinch of dried oregano

sea salt and black pepper (if using chicken jelly stock cubes, you probably won't need salt)

leaves from 1 bunch of coriander, very finely chopped

leaves from 1 bunch of flat leaf parsley, very finely chopped

This winter favourite takes a little time but is so worth the effort. It's based on a traditional Italian wedding soup that Ina Garten introduced me to. Lots of ingredients, I know – but batch it.

Firstly prepare the meatballs. Start by heating 1 tablespoon of the olive oil in a casserole over a medium heat. Add the shallot, dried herbs and mushrooms and cook until the mushrooms are browned. Add the splash of wine and sauté until the pan is dry. Now reduce the heat and add the garlic, just for a minute. Set aside in a bowl to cool.

Tip both types of minced meat into a large bowl, breaking it up gently with a fork. Very lightly mix in the cooled sautéed mixture until combined, taking care not to overwork it, or the meatballs will not be light. Add the parsley and season generously. Roll the mixture gently into little balls, about 3cm (1¼ inches) in diameter. Put them on a plate and set aside in the fridge for 10–30 minutes, if you have time. This will help them to stay together in the pan.

In the same casserole pan, add the remaining 1 tablespoon of olive oil and sauté the onions, celery and carrot until tender. Scrape into a bowl, leaving behind as much oil in the pan as possible.

Take the meatballs out of the fridge and, in the same pan over medium-high heat, brown them all over for 3–4 minutes. Now return the onion mixture, add the tomatoes, pour in the stock, add the oregano and bring to the boil. Immediately reduce the heat to a gentle simmer until the meatballs are cooked through, but still tender; this should take 12 minutes.

Taste and add more stock and seasoning if needed and stir in the herbs to serve.

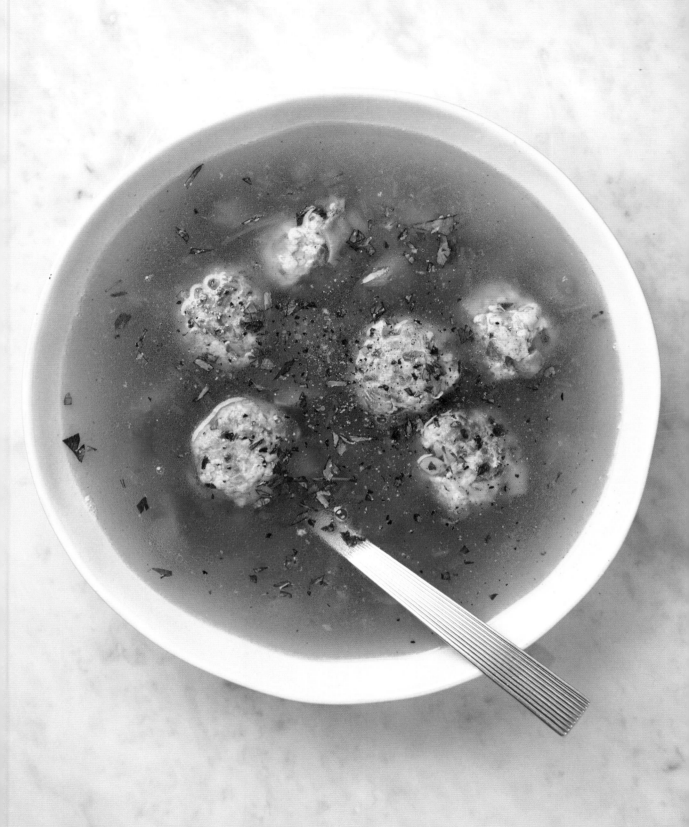

Tex Mex

400g (14oz) chicken breast or leftover cooked chicken

1–1.5 litres (4–6 cups) good chicken stock

1 tablespoon groundnut oil

1 large onion, finely chopped

½ teaspoon dried oregano

½ teaspoon ground cumin

200g (1 cup) green tomatoes (or yellow), chopped

2 large green mild chillies, sliced

2 garlic cloves, crushed

400g (14oz) can chickpeas, drained and rinsed

juice of 1 lime, plus lime wedges to serve

sea salt and black pepper

2 radishes, finely sliced

100g (3½oz) coriander, leaves separated and chopped

1 ripe avocado, sliced

Another great use for leftover chicken, but interchange with any bean or tofu if you're veggie and use good vegetable stock instead. My kids adore this served with purple corn chips which you can add in for guests or family sides for a quick weekend lunch.

If you're using raw chicken, poach it in a shallow pan in the chicken stock for 10–15 minutes (depending on the size) until cooked through, but still tender. Reserve the stock and cut the chicken into cubes. If you are using leftover cooked chicken, cut it into little cubes or shred it.

Heat the oil in a saucepan over a medium heat, adding the onion, oregano and cumin, and sauté until the onion is translucent but not brown. Add the green tomatoes, 1 of the chillies and the garlic and sauté for 2 minutes. Now pour in 1 litre (4 cups) of the reserved stock, add the chicken and chickpeas and bring to the boil. Squeeze in the lime juice. Adjust salt and pepper to taste, and add more stock if liked.

Pour into bowls; I like a shallow bowl so there is space to decorate, and garnish with the lime wedges, radishes, the remaining green chilli, the coriander and avocado.

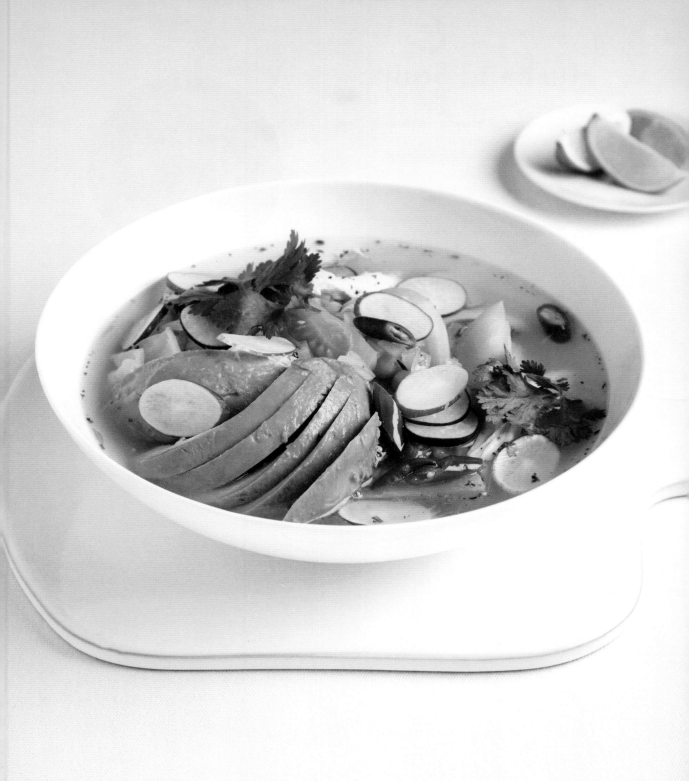

Husband Soup

The most tedious part of this recipe is peeling and slicing the onions finely, so I always casually ask my husband to do this while I act very busy...You can replace the beef with kidney beans for a veggie version too.

Serves 4

1 tablespoon unsalted butter

1 tablespoon olive oil

9 large onions, finely sliced

1 bay leaf (dried is fine)

100ml (scant ½ cup) good brandy

100ml (scant ½ cup) white wine

1.5 litres (6 cups) good beef stock (from the chilled cabinet in the supermarket)

600g (1lb 5oz) sliced leftover beef fillet

leaves from 1 bunch of flat leaf parsley, roughly chopped

2 tablespoons finely grated pecorino cheese

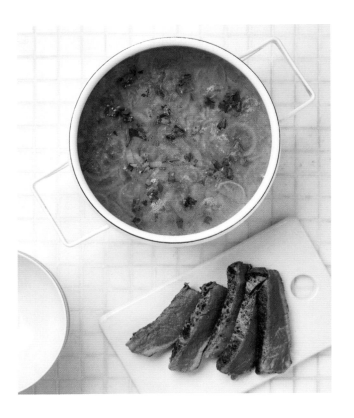

Heat the butter and oil in a large saucepan over a medium heat and add the onions all in one go. Just slowly stir, stir, stir them until – after about 15 minutes – they turn very soft and brown. If you rush this and they don't brown beautifully, it won't wow you.

Deglaze the pan with the brandy and wine, scraping the base of the pan to get off all the good browned bits, then simply add the stock. Return to the boil and simmer gently, lid off, for another 10 minutes.

Add the slices of beef and, once they are piping hot, serve in big bowls, sprinkled with parsley and pecorino.

My Seafood Bouillabaisse

Chop and change in the seafood that you love. The trick is to intensify the flavour with good stock and to cook the shellfish with the shell on, which also makes for a messier and lovelier meal. Add chunks of wholemeal bread for your family or guests.

Serves 4

1 tablespoon olive oil

2 leeks, sliced

6 tomatoes, chopped

1 red pepper, chopped

1 fennel bulb, sliced, or to taste

pinch of finely grated unwaxed orange zest

½ thyme sprig

1 bay leaf

1 garlic clove, crushed

1–1.5 litres (4–6 cups) good fish stock

150g (5½oz) monkfish, cubed

125g (4½oz) salmon, cubed

150g (5½oz) prawns, shells on

250g (9oz) mussels, shells on, cleaned

pinch of saffron threads

juice of 1 lemon, plus 1 lemon, cut into wedges

sea salt and black pepper

small handful of tarragon leaves, chopped

handful of flat leaf parsley leaves, chopped

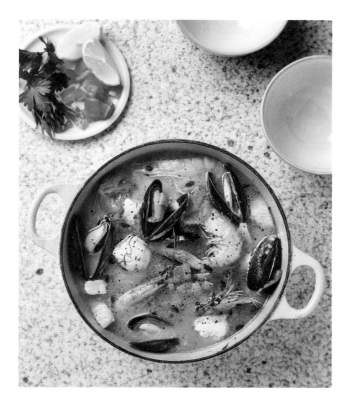

Heat the olive oil in a large saucepan over a medium heat, add the leeks and cook for a few minutes until translucent but not brown. Add the tomatoes and red pepper and sauté gently for 4 minutes. Now add the fennel, orange zest, thyme, bay leaf and garlic and 1 litre (4 cups) of the stock.

Increase the heat to high, then reduce to a simmer. Add all the seafood and simmer very gently until it is firm, be careful not to overcook. Stir in the saffron and lemon juice. Taste and adjust the seasoning.

Sprinkle with the herbs and serve with lemon wedges on the side.

4.
SALADS

I hope you love some of my favourite salads included in this chapter. The varieties are just endless, so I've included a section on how to build a salad the Louise Parker way. Please consider the four building blocks when you're thinking of making a salad: flavour, texture, crunch and variety. And use the very best ingredients you can afford. There are winter options and summer options here, and use warm protein on days when you need a little more comfort.

Play around with different dressings – see my 8 dressings on pages 121–3 to transform the same chicken salad. And promise me you won't serve yourself some Iceberg lettuce and dry chicken in a pot; that is not a salad, it's a punishment meal (plus it reeks of the 1980s: great for many things, not for food). Love flavour – and remember that every meal is meant to be really enjoyed.

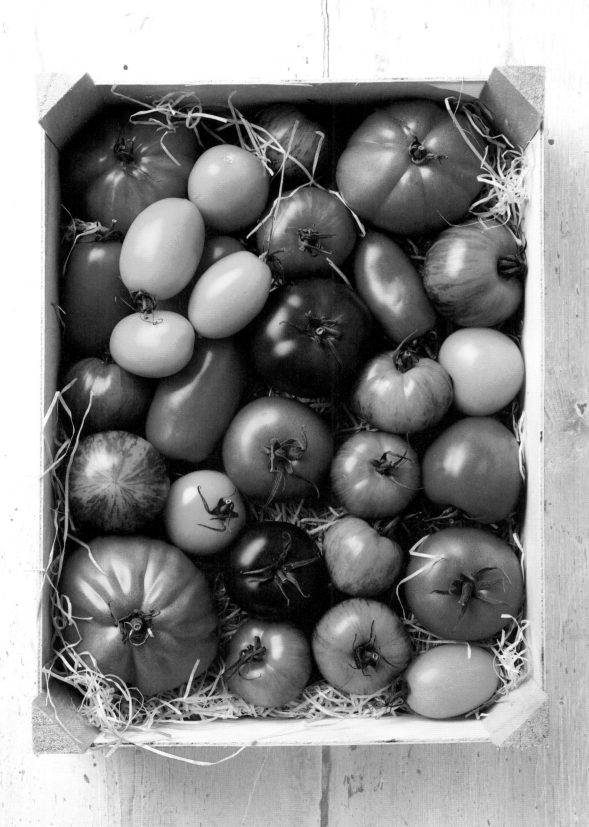

HOW TO BUILD A SALAD

GO BIG, GO GREEN

Every salad needs a base and it's usually a green vegetable or salad leaves. Think beyond iceberg lettuce and try every leaf imaginable, or include raw and al dente veggies.

salad leaves ★ lower-GI roasted vegetables ★ raw veggies ★ blanched veg from leftovers

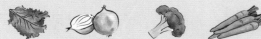

LOVE FLAVOUR & TEXTURE

Now it's time to add another layer of flavour to your salad. Think about classic combinations of ingredients, mix cooked and raw, add splashes of colour and mix up textures.

peas & beans ★ tomatoes & peppers ★ avocados ★ onions ★ radishes

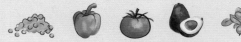

WHERE'S THE PROTEIN?

The list of protein sources is endless and, as with the veggies, try your salads with hot and cold variations. Vary them and experiment.

eggs ★ soy protein ★ fish ★ pulses & legumes ★ lower-fat cheese ★ meats

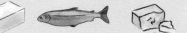

DRESS TO IMPRESS

The last two steps are when you take a 'diet' salad to a delicious salad. Your dressing is also where you add in healthy fat, zing and flavour. See pages 121–3 for 8 ways to build a dressing. Always add your dressing right before you eat.

See pages 121–3

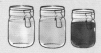

FLAVOUR, GARNISH & TEXTURE

The last part is where you really get to show off. Adding a little extra crunch, colour, spice and zing takes an 8/10 salad to 10/10. Ditch croutons in favour of a few toasted nuts, seeds, sliced chilli or some extra fresh herbs. Add just before serving.

seeds ★ toasted nuts ★ fresh herbs ★ chilli ★ citrus fruits

Simple Saigon

This light fragrant salad is perfect for a light lunch and, as all the ingredients are firm, keeps for a day or so, making a great lunchbox for the following day. (Just don't add the dressing if you are going to keep it for another day.) I love this recipe with prawns, leftover turkey or calamari, often buying those ready cooked, so I can assemble this salad in a matter of minutes after a long day.

Serves 4

FOR THE SALAD

4 x 150g (5½oz) skinless chicken breasts, cooked

½ red cabbage, shredded

½ Savoy cabbage, shredded

12 radishes, finely sliced

3 spring onions, cut in thirds lengthways

good handful of coriander leaves

good handful of Thai basil leaves

good handful of mint leaves

4 tablespoons peanuts, skin on

4 mild red chillies, finely chopped

FOR THE DRESSING

½ teaspoon peeled and finely chopped fresh root ginger (or ginger purée)

1 garlic clove, finely chopped

juice and finely grated zest of 2 unwaxed limes

pinch of stevia, to taste

1 teaspoon rice wine vinegar

½ teaspoon fish sauce

1 tablespoon groundnut oil

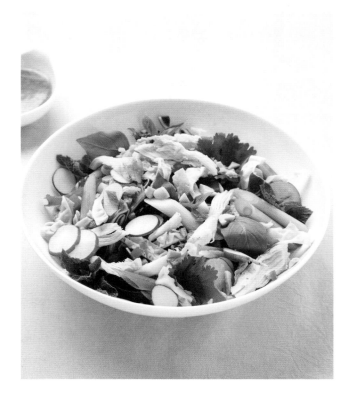

Tear the cooked chicken into bite-sized pieces. Build the salad on a platter with the cabbage, radishes, spring onions, and whole leaves of coriander, basil and mint.

To make the dressing, simply combine all the ingredients in a bowl and whisk.

Add the dressing and chicken to the salad and toss well to ensure everything is evenly coated (don't add the dressing if making this in advance).

Chop the peanuts and toss in a hot wok just until they begin to brown, then remove from the heat.

Top the salad with the chillies to taste and the hot toasted peanuts.

Miso, Tahini & Tofu ⓥ

Serves 4

FOR THE SALAD

1 tablespoon white sesame seeds

2 teaspoons black sesame seeds

200g (7oz) baby asparagus spears

200g (7oz) green beans

200g (7oz) tenderstem broccoli

1 tablespoon groundnut oil

6 large or 12 small oyster mushrooms, thickly sliced

50–100ml (¼–½ cup) vegetable stock

2 chicory heads, very finely sliced

½ small red onion, very finely sliced

1 red chilli, finely chopped

good handful of coriander leaves, finely chopped

small handful of mint leaves, finely chopped

700g (1lb 9oz) firm smoked tofu, cut into thick slices

1 teaspoon sesame oil

FOR THE DRESSING

1 quantity Tahini and Miso dressing (see page 121)

I go heavy on the mushrooms here as I adore them, but simply swap out any ingredients that you don't love. I often serve this salad with sliced chargrilled steak, which works beautifully with the tahini dressing.

Begin by toasting the sesame seeds in a dry frying pan over a medium heat until they turn ever so slightly golden and smell toasty. Set aside to cool. Cut the asparagus, beans and broccoli into equal-sized pieces.

Using the same pan, heat ½ tablespoon of the groundnut oil over a medium-high heat. Fry the mushrooms for 2 minutes on each side until they are browned. Remove and set aside.

Now add the remaining ½ tablespoon of groundnut oil and stir-fry the asparagus, beans and broccoli, adding enough vegetable stock to steam-fry until they are cooked, but still all dente. Set aside to cool.

Arrange the chicory, onion, chilli, coriander and mint on a platter.

Finally, brush the tofu slices with the sesame oil, and griddle on a non-stick griddle pan for 1 minute on each side, until they are browned and stripy.

To assemble, just layer the cooled stir-fried veggies and mushrooms over the chopped salad, arrange the tofu on top, drizzle with the dressing and sprinkle with the toasted sesame seeds to serve.

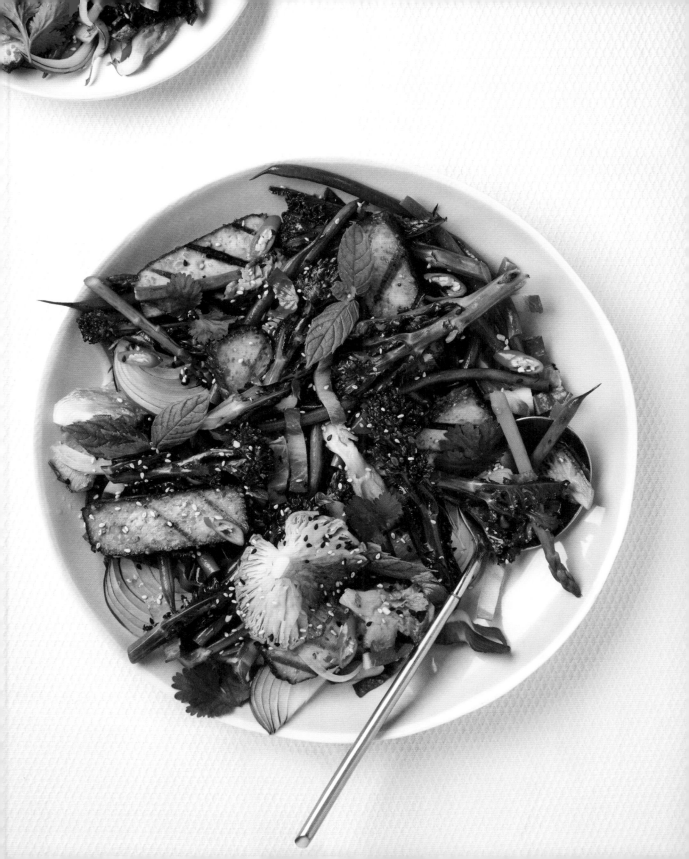

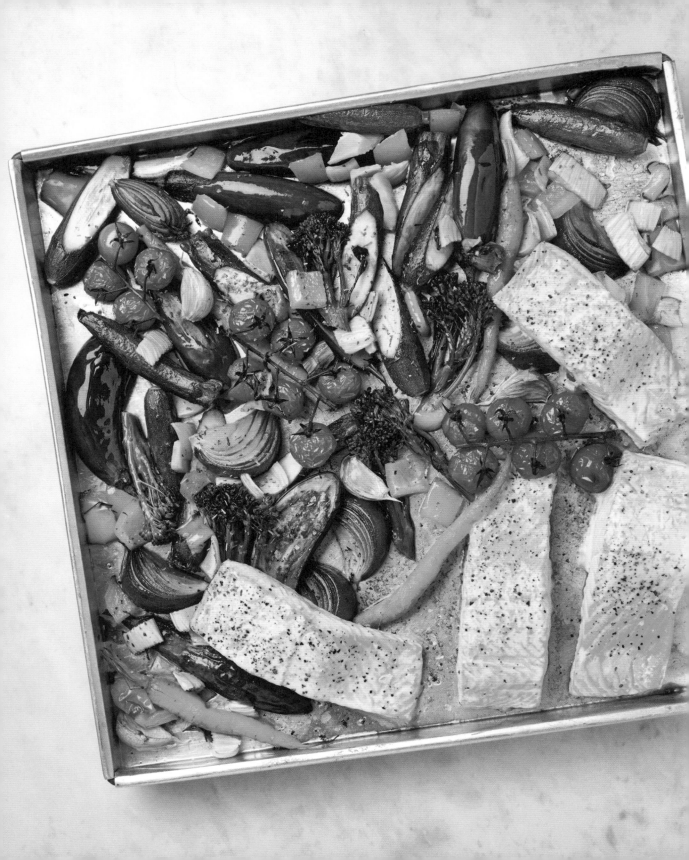

Warm Winter Roast

Serves 4

FOR THE SALAD

4 baby aubergines,
halved lengthways

8 baby courgettes, halved lengthways

4 baby carrots, halved lengthways

300g (10½oz) tenderstem broccoli,
in small florets

2 red onions, quartered

400g (2 cups) cherry tomatoes

1 yellow pepper, cut into chunks

1 small fennel bulb, chopped

2 tablespoons olive oil

1 tablespoon aged balsamic vinegar

½ teaspoon dried oregano

sea salt and black pepper

4 garlic cloves, skin on

4 x 150g (5½oz) salmon fillets

juice of ½ orange

150g (6 packed cups) rocket

150g (6 packed cups) spinach leaves

50g (½ cup) hazelnuts,
toasted and chopped

FOR THE DRESSING

2 tablespoon olive oil

juice of 1 orange

Roasting the veggies for this salad intensifies the flavours and offers a gloriously warming and comforting salad when the last thing you want is cold leaves. If making any swaps, avoid higher-GI veggies such as butternut, parsnip and potato until you're into the Lifestyle Phase.

Preheat the oven to 240°C/475°F/Gas Mark 9.

Prepare the vegetables and toss in the olive oil, balsamic vinegar, dried oregano, seasoning and garlic. Roast in the top of the oven for 35 minutes until the veggies begin to brown; do keep an eye on them as you don't want them to burn.

Meanwhile, drench the salmon fillets in the orange juice, season and bake in the bottom half of the oven for 10 minutes, giving the veggies a quick check and a toss as you do so.

Meanwhile, assemble the rocket and spinach on a platter. Take the vegetables out of the oven and remove the garlic cloves; discard all but 1 of these (for the dressing).

Prepare the dressing by squeezing the soft garlic clove out of its skin into a cup and whisking it with the olive oil, orange juice and seasoning. Pour over the roasted vegetables and give them a quick toss.

Arrange the roasted vegetables on the bed of leaves, placing the salmon fillets on top, and sprinkle with the hazelnuts to serve.

Celery & Apple Refresher (Vg)

Gorgeously zingy and fresh, this works as a light meal, or I often use it as a side with a good piece of grilled salmon. It's great for barbecues too.

Serves 4

2 unwaxed oranges

juice of 1–2 lemons

1 tablespoon olive oil

sea salt and black pepper

2 cucumbers, deseeded and cut into batons

1 fennel bulb, finely sliced lengthways

1 green apple, peeled, cored and cut into matchsticks

2 celery sticks, cut into matchsticks, plus celery leaves to serve

4 tablespoons pumpkin seeds

Remove ½ teaspoon of the orange zest with a zester and finely chop it. Set aside. Now peel the oranges completely, removing all the white pith, then slice them into rounds. Arrange around the edges of a serving plate.

Whisk together the lemon juice, olive oil, orange zest and seasoning.

In a bowl, toss together the cucumbers, fennel, apple and celery with the lemony dressing. Pile these in the middle of the orange slices.

Sprinkle with the celery leaves (or use parsley leaves, if there weren't any celery leaves on the bunch).

Toast the pumpkin seeds in a dry frying pan and scatter on top to serve.

Cauliflower & Feta (V)

I always double up on roasted cauliflower when making this, so I have leftovers for salads. This also works with paprika or any Middle Eastern herb mix.

Serves 4

1 large cauliflower, cut into florets

2 tablespoons good olive oil, plus 1 teaspoon to fry the rosemary

1 tablespoon finely chopped rosemary leaves, plus 1 tablespoon mini rosemary sprigs

sea salt and black pepper

juice of 2 lemons, plus ½ teaspoon finely grated unwaxed lemon zest

400g (14oz) can butter beans, drained and rinsed

200g (8 packed cups) rocket

100g (1 cup) feta, crumbled

Preheat the oven to 240°C/475°F/Gas Mark 9.

Put the cauliflower on a baking tray, toss with half the olive oil and the rosemary, season well, then roast in the middle of the oven for 30 minutes. Remove and allow to cool a little. Whisk together the other 1 tablespoon of olive oil with the lemon juice and zest.

While the cauliflower is still warm, combine it with the beans. Toss both in the dressing and lay on a bed of the rocket on a platter.

Fry the rosemary sprigs in the remaining olive oil for 90 seconds. Finish the salad by crumbling over the feta cheese and adding the fried rosemary.

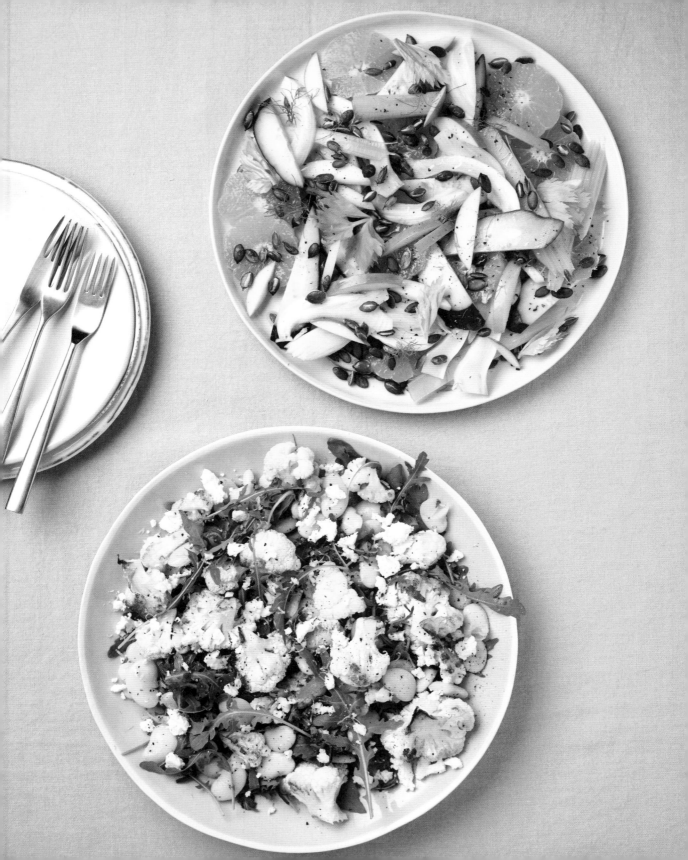

Roquefort, Pear & Chicory Salad

Serves 4

4 pears, skin on, cored and halved

150g (5½oz) Roquefort cheese

8 slices prosciutto, visible fat removed

2 heads of red chicory

2 heads of white chicory

100g (¾ cup) pomegranate seeds

16 walnuts, chopped and toasted

4 tablespoons Classic French Dressing
(see page 122)

This is lower in protein than most of my meals, so it's best suited for a light evening meal when you want something quick and full of flavour, but bear in mind it's not as filling as most of my recipes.

Preheat the oven to 200°C/400°F/Gas Mark 6.

First, prepare the pears and divide the Roquefort cheese evenly between the halves, placing a little dollop in the centre of each pear half. Now take a piece of prosciutto, wrap it round each half and pop on a baking tray. Bake in the oven for 20 minutes until the prosciutto crisps nicely.

Prepare the simple salad by finely slicing the heads of chicory lengthways. Arrange the leaves on a plate, with the baked pears, and top with the pomegranate seeds and toasted walnuts, which I like to chop before toasting so that you've a bit of crunch in each mouthful.

Dress with the French dressing and serve.

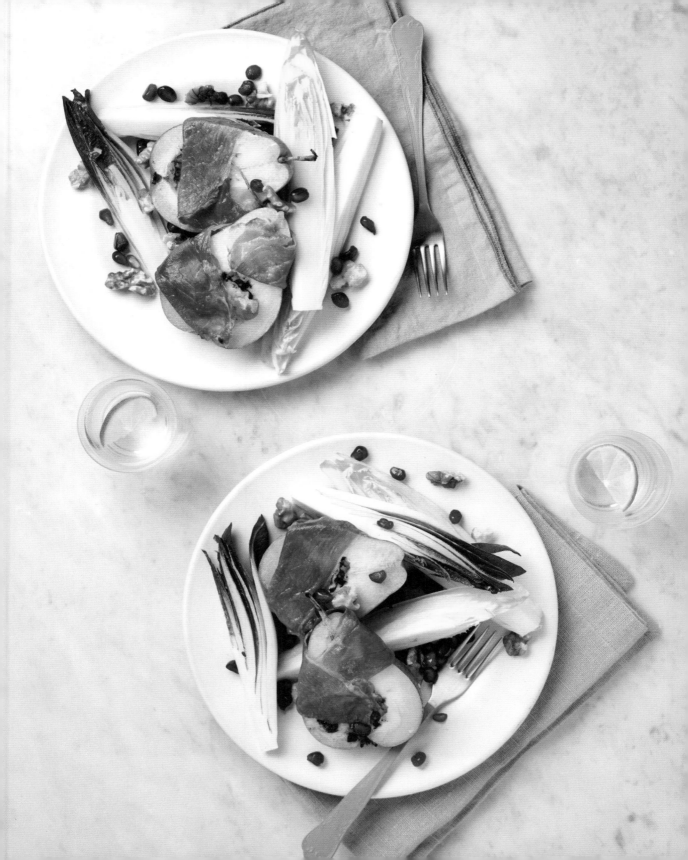

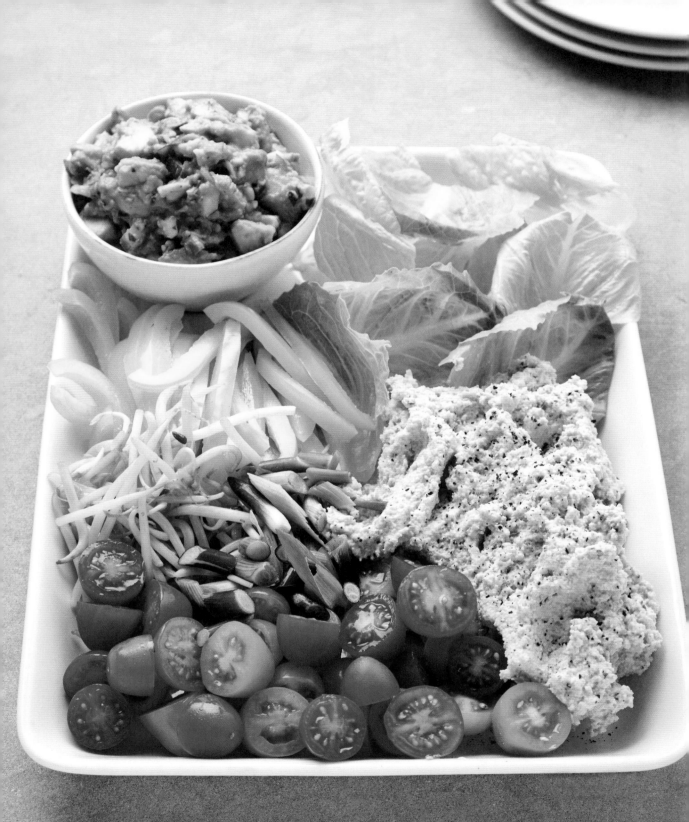

Vegan Mex (Vg)

Serves 4

FOR THE SALAD BASE

2 Romaine lettuces, leaves torn

200g (1 cup) cherry tomatoes, halved

2 spring onions, chopped into strips

2 yellow peppers, finely sliced

150g (1½ cups) beansprouts

FOR THE 'MEAT'

600g (1lb 5oz) firm tofu, roughly chopped

10–12 artichoke hearts

leaves from 1 large bunch of flat leaf parsley, chopped

juice of 3 limes

1 teaspoon sea salt

FOR THE GUACAMOLE

2 ripe avocados

juice of 2 limes

leaves from 1 large bunch of coriander, chopped

2 green chillies, finely chopped, or to taste

½ red onion, finely chopped

sea salt and black pepper

dash of green Tabasco sauce, to taste

This dish comes courtesy of Alejandra, who is so clever at concocting vegan dishes that have real zing. The artichoke works so well with the tofu. Adjust the chilli and lime to taste

Prepare the base of the salad, arranging all the prepared vegetables on a platter with the beansprouts and leaves.

Transfer all the ingredients for the 'meat' mixture to a food processor and pulse until it becomes smooth-ish, but still with a few bits to chew on. Add to the salad serving dish.

To make the guacamole, simply combine all the ingredients in a bowl and give it a really good mash with a fork; I like mine a little chunky. Taste for chilli and seasoning and adjust as necessary. Add to the salad and tofu mixture to serve.

My Favourite Tabbouleh ⓥ

Serves 4

FOR THE SALAD

leaves from 1 large bunch
of coriander

leaves from 1 large bunch
of flat leaf parsley

leaves from 1 large bunch of mint

12 tomatoes, deseeded and chopped

400g (14oz) can chickpeas,
skinned if you have time

sea salt and black pepper

1 tablespoon za'atar

200g (7oz) haloumi cheese, sliced

125g (4½oz) pomegranate seeds

FOR THE DRESSING

juice of 2 lemons, plus ½ teaspoon
finely grated unwaxed lemon zest

2 tablespoons olive oil

½ teaspoon chopped mint leaves

I'm obsessed with tabbouleh and love nothing more than the smell that comes from chopping great big handfuls of fresh herbs. This is so full of goodness and can easily be adapted. Increase the amount of chickpeas if haloumi is not your thing.

Finely chop all the herbs: I use a huge knife and board, combine all the herbs together and just chop away for a couple of minutes. Deseed the tomatoes (or just use cherry tomatoes cut in half if you're in a hurry) and simply combine all the herbs, tomatoes and chickpeas together in a bowl. Give it a good stir and taste for seasoning. It requires more salt and pepper than you think, but adjust depending on whether you are serving it with some beans or meat, or salty cheese as I am here (in which case, use less).

Put the za'atar on a flat plate and dab in each side of the sliced haloumi, before popping on a hot non-stick griddle pan, giving each side about 45 seconds or until it is beautifully brown and stripy.

Prepare the dressing by whisking all the ingredients together. Mix with the herbs and chickpeas in the mixing bowl.

Serve the griddled haloumi on top of the salad and sprinkle with the pomegranate seeds.

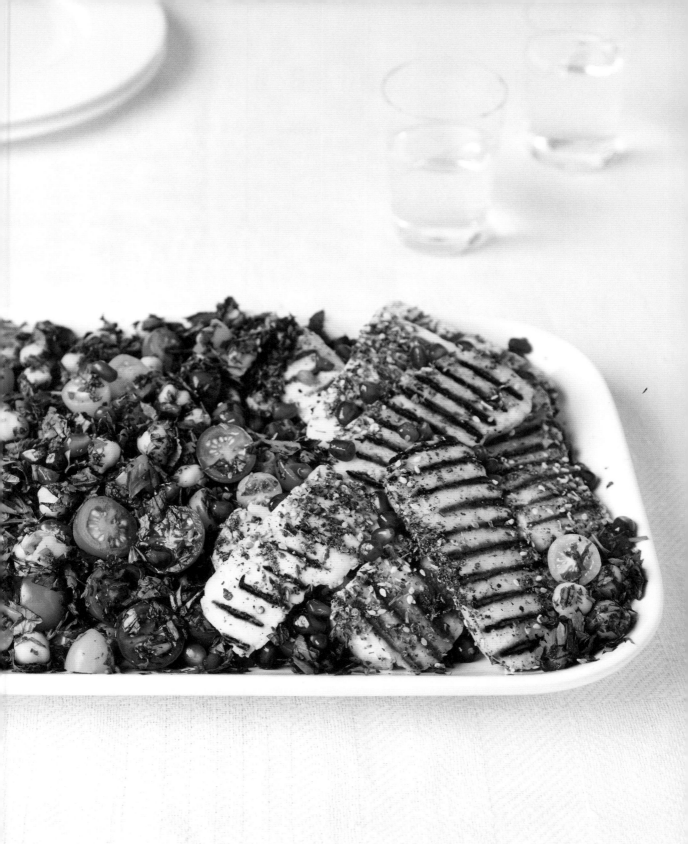

Black & White Beluga Salad

Serves 4

400g (14oz) ready-cooked beluga lentils

2–3 tablespoons aged balsamic vinegar, plus extra to serve

2 tablespoons capers, drained and rinsed, plus extra to serve

1 tablespoon good pesto

sea salt and black pepper

leaves from 1 large bunch of flat leaf parsley, chopped

leaves from 1 large bunch of basil, chopped

1 spring onion, finely sliced

200g (1 cup) cherry tomatoes

1 tablespoons pine nuts

150g (5½oz) slice of soft goats' cheese

heads of 2–3 red chicory (optional)

This recipe is super-fast and filling, and it's great with leftover torn chicken. Again, if you don't like goats' cheese, swap in another – don't be a slave to the recipe. I cheat and use ready cooked beluga lentils, which I always have in my store cupboard.

Place the lentils, balsamic vinegar, capers, pesto, sea salt, black pepper, herbs, spring onion and tomatoes in a bowl and combine everything together well.

Fry the pine nuts in a dry frying pan over a medium heat until they turn a shade darker and smell toasted, then tip out on to a plate.

Crumble the goats' cheese on top of the salad and sprinkle over the toasted pine nuts.

Serve alongside – or inside – chicory leaves, with extra balsamic, chilli and capers, if liked.

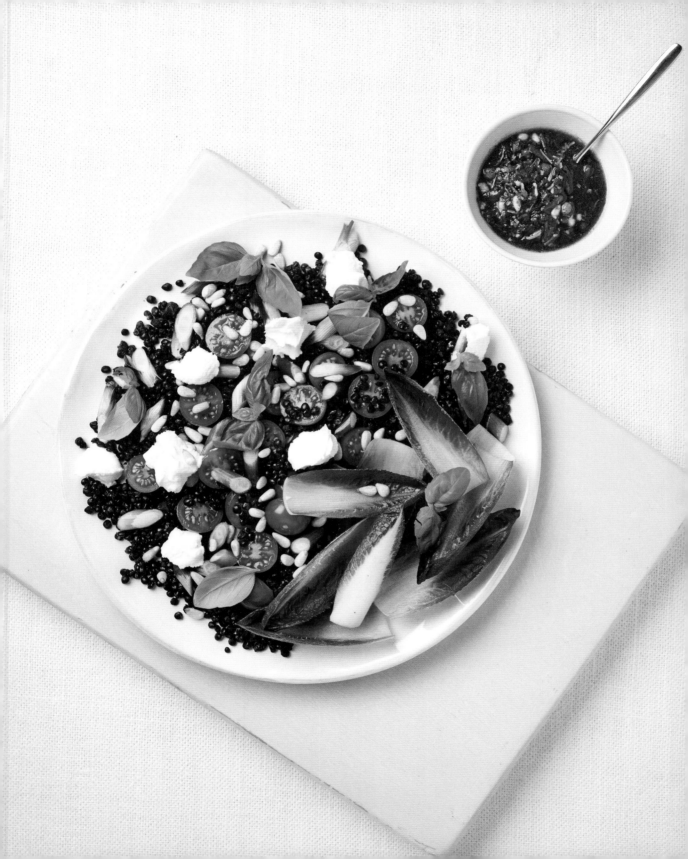

My ChopChop Salad

Serves 4

2 avocados

juice of 1 lime

200g (1½ cups) frozen
edamame beans

leaves from 1 large bunch of
coriander, finely chopped

leaves from 1 large bunch of flat leaf
parsley, finely chopped

leaves from 1 large bunch of mint,
finely chopped, plus extra to garnish

400g (2 cups) cherry tomatoes,
finely chopped

1 cucumber, deseeded and
finely chopped

4 Little Gem lettuces, finely chopped

2 yellow peppers, finely chopped

3 ready-cooked chicken breasts,
chopped

sea salt and black pepper

Everything tastes better chopped up and this is perhaps my favourite salad. It relies on good, ripe avocados – I store mine in a brown paper bag or newspaper in the cupboard until perfectly ripe. You can add some variety by swapping one of the chicken breasts for two boiled eggs.

Finely chop the avocados and drench with the lime juice to keep them green.

Defrost the edamame by pouring boiling water on them and set aside while you continue chopping.

Mix the herbs together in a large bowl. Add all the remaining ingredients, including the chopped avocados and drained edamame beans. Stir gently to combine and then check the seasoning before arranging on a platter. Serve garnished with the extra mint leaves.

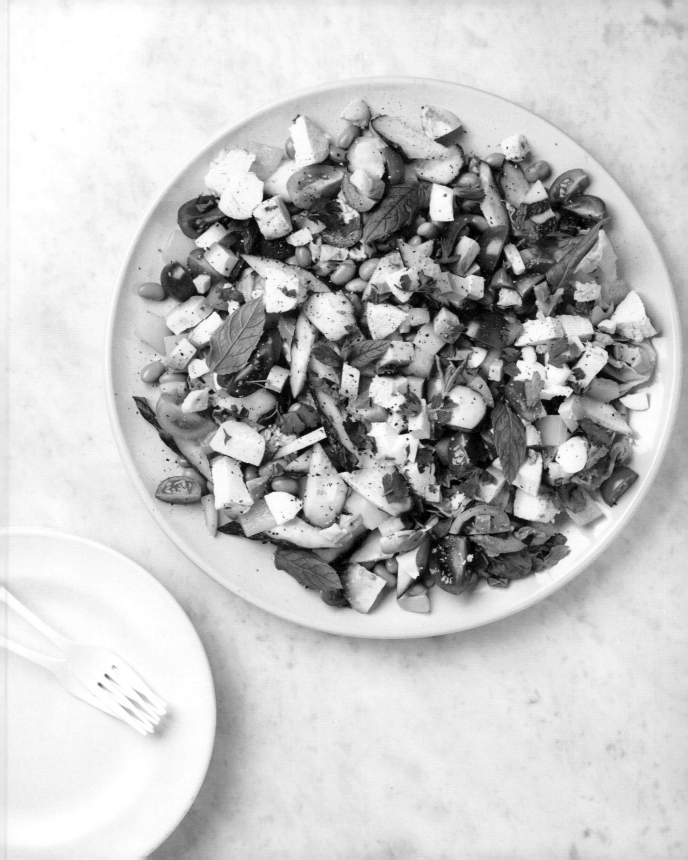

HOW TO BUILD A DRESSING

All my salad dressings are balanced and I suggest a serving of 2 tablespoons for each salad.
You can always add more citrus or vinegar to taste, too. These should all keep in a screwtop
jar in the fridge for up to 3 days

1 PART HEALTHY FAT

Every dressing needs one part healthy fat, but watch your portions here as fats do pack a calorific punch.
Buy the best quality oils you can and, if you want to be lean, forget those TV-chef-style huge glugs of olive oil.

olive oil ★ sesame oil ★ walnut oil ★ groundnut oil ★ hazelnut oil

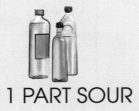

1 PART SOUR

Next you need to add some zing to your base. I usually work to a 1:1 ratio with the fat but you can experiment with a little
more or less sour to taste. As with wines, you can notice a huge difference if you spend a little more on your vinegars.

**apple cider vinegar ★ balsamic vinegar ★ champagne vinegar ★ red wine or white wine vinegars
★ lemon, lime or orange juices & zest**

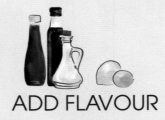

ADD FLAVOUR

In this last part you get to really play around with all sorts of flavours. Experiment and try new combinations but also
don't be afraid of making a simple French dressing. Done well, it will still take your breath away.

**salt & pepper ★ raw or roasted garlic ★ miso paste ★ herbs ★ spices ★ wasabi or horseradish
★ chilli ★ mustards (these help to emulsify a dressing)**

① Homemade Pesto

Serves 4

25g (¼ cup) walnut pieces, toasted

25g (¼ cup) pine nuts

25g (¼ cup) grated Parmesan

100g (3½oz) basil leaves

¼ garlic clove

pinch of finely grated unwaxed lemon zest

juice of 2 lemons

sea salt and black pepper

Add all the ingredients to a mini blender and whizz until smooth (or cheat with 1 part good shop-bought pesto and 2 parts lemon juice).

② Tarragon Mayo ⓥ

Serves 4

5 teaspoons full-fat mayonnaise

5 teaspoons 0% Greek yogurt

10 teaspoons lemon juice

1 teaspoon Dijon mustard

1 teaspoon chopped tarragon leaves

sea salt and black pepper

Whisk all the ingredients together with a fork, or blend for a more intense tarragon flavour.

③ Tahini & Miso ⓥg

Serves 4

1 tablespoon tahini

1 tablespoon sweet white miso

1 tablespoon lemon juice

1 tablespoon sesame oil

2 tablespoons water

1cm (½ inch) fresh root ginger, peeled and finely grated, or to taste

Combine all the ingredients in a mini blender and whizz for 1 minute.

④ Passion Fruit ⓥg

Serves 4

8 teaspoons passion fruit pulp

8 teaspoons olive oil

4 teaspoons lime juice

sea salt and black pepper

Sieve the passion fruit pulp into a bowl to remove the seeds. Add the remaining ingredients and whisk with a fork. Taste for seasoning and adjust.

⑤ Walnut Vinaigrette ⓥg

Serves 4

6 teaspoons chopped walnuts, toasted

6 teaspoons walnut oil

12 teaspoons balsamic vinegar

2 teaspoons Dijon mustard

sea salt and black pepper

Shake together all the ingredients in a screwtop jar until combined.

⑥ Classic French ⓥg

Serves 4

8 teaspoons champagne vinegar

8 teaspoons good olive oil

4 teaspoons Dijon mustard

crushed or very finely chopped garlic, to taste

sea salt and black pepper

Combine all the ingredients in a mini blender and whizz for 1 minute.

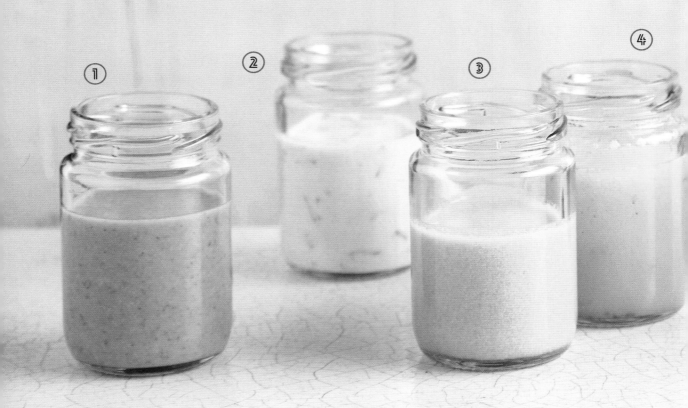

⑦ Satay Chilli ⓥg

Serves 4

2 tablespoons sugar-free peanut butter

2 tablespoons sesame oil

4 tablespoons lime juice

1 garlic clove, crushed or very finely chopped, or to taste

½ red chilli, finely chopped, or to taste

sea salt and black pepper

Add the peanut butter, sesame oil and lime juice to a mini blender and whizz, adding the garlic, chilli and salt and pepper a little at a time, to taste.

⑧ Green Goddess ⓥ

Serves 4

15g (¾ packed cup) basil

15g (¾ packed cup) tarragon

15g (¾ packed cup) flat leaf parsley

15g (¾ packed cup) dill

3½ tablespoons full-fat Greek yogurt

3 tablespoons olive oil

juice of ½ lemon

sea salt and black pepper

Combine all the ingredients except the salt and pepper in a mini blender. Check the seasoning, then slowly add salt and pepper, to taste.

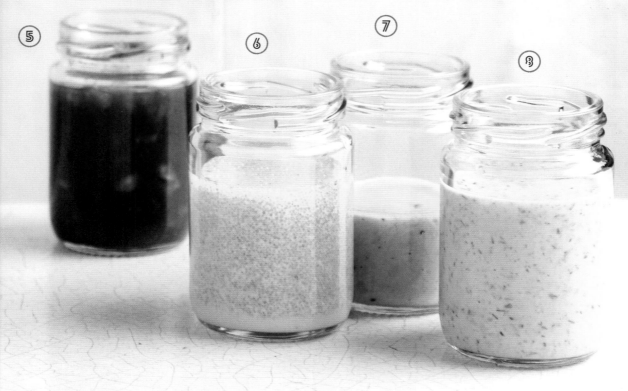

5

MAINS

As we're all short on time, I've included some speedier, simpler meals in this section, as well as others that take a little bit longer and require a longer list of ingredients. Don't be put off those, because once your store cupboard is prepped, they'll be so much easier to whizz together than you think (and it gives you a great excuse to buy lots of lovely kitchen storage vessels).

Some recipes in this section are great for batch-cooking and freezing, others perfect for midweek dinners when you only have a few minutes to spend in the kitchen, and I've included vegetarian and vegan options too, because you asked and I listened… I hope you enjoy them as much as we do. These mains are intended to be eaten either for lunch or supper, so swap them around depending on the seasons, your appetite, your schedule, the weather and your mood.

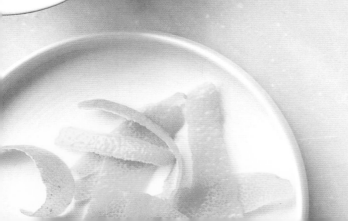

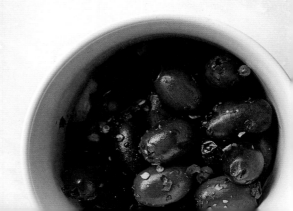

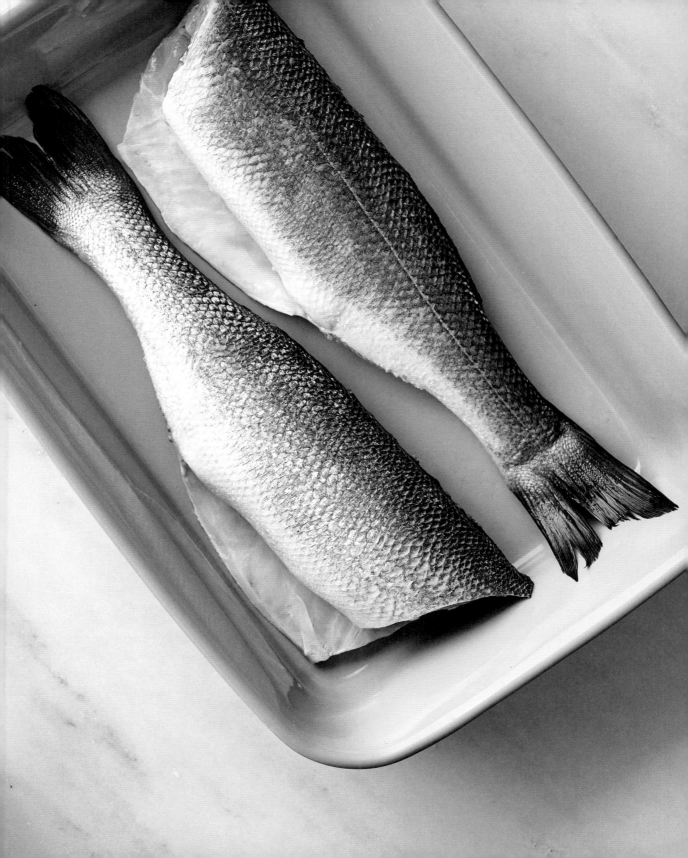

GanGan's Pot Roast

Serves 8 (with leftovers)

2kg (4lb 8oz) joint of silverside or topside of beef

1 tablespoon sea salt

1 tablespoon black pepper

1 teaspoon English mustard powder

½ tablespoon very finely chopped rosemary leaves

2 tablespoons wholemeal flour

3½ tablespoons unsalted butter

2 tablespoons olive oil

4 carrots, thickly sliced at an angle

6 celery sticks, thickly sliced at an angle

12 shallots, peeled

2 thyme sprigs

200ml (scant 1 cup) red wine

100ml (scant ½ cup) brandy

2 x 400g (14oz) cans cherry tomatoes

100ml (scant ½ cup) water

1 chicken jelly stock cube

1 bouquet garni

1 whole garlic bulb, halved

1 tablespoon Worcestershire sauce

16 baby courgettes, halved

2 teaspoons cornflour

When we lived in Sussex I'd make this after the Friday school run, just in time for hungry friends from London to visit. It's wonderful the next day too.

Preheat the oven to 160°C/325°F/Gas Mark 3.

Pat the joint dry with kitchen paper, then rub well with the salt and pepper. Mix the mustard, rosemary and flour on a flat plate and roll the meat in the mixture until lightly covered.

Heat the butter and half the oil in a large casserole over a medium-high heat and seal each side of the joint. Remove and set aside.

Add the remaining oil, carrots, celery, shallots and thyme and stir for 10 minutes until the vegetables soften. Add the wine and brandy and increase the heat for 2 minutes. Reduce the heat to medium and throw in the tomatoes, water, stock cube, bouquet garni, garlic and Worcestershire sauce. Return the beef to the dish, bring to the boil, put the lid on, then put in the oven for 1 hour.

Turn the joint and reduce the oven temperature to 150°C/300°F/Gas Mark 2. Leave in the oven, covered, for 1½ hours.

Remove the joint from the dish, cover in foil and leave for 20 minutes to rest before carving.

Skim as much fat as possible from the sauce, discarding the thyme sticks and garlic bulbs. Reduce over a low heat for 15 minutes. Once reduced, put half of the sauce in a blender, whizz until smooth, then return it to the dish. Add the courgettes and simmer for 5 minutes until they're cooked but still a little firm. Mix the cornflour in a little water, then mix into a cup of the sauce, before returning to the pan. Stir until the sauce thickens beautifully and check the seasoning.

Serve the courgettes and sauce in large bowls, with 2–3 thick slices of beef per person.

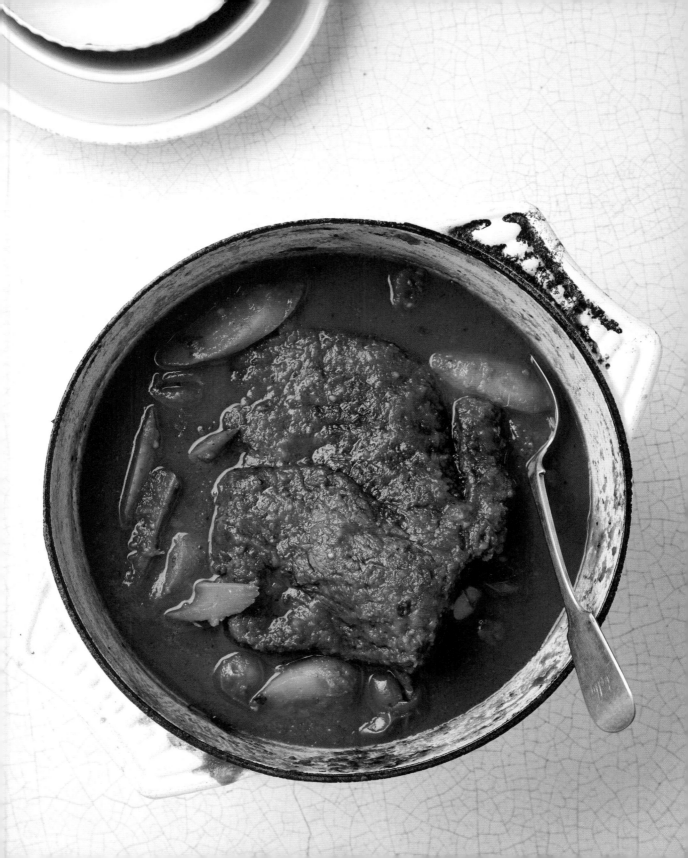

Lemon Sole & Cauliflower Cream

The trick for cauliflower cream is a dash of cream and generous seasoning. Sprinkle with a little Parmesan if you like. This is a wonderful combination with the lemon sole, although I often serve it with sea bass, steak or sausages too. Kids love it.

Serves 4

FOR THE CAULIFLOWER CREAM

1 cauliflower

50ml (scant ¼ cup) single cream

100–200ml (½–¾ cup) milk

sea salt and black pepper

FOR THE SOLE

3½ tablespoons unsalted butter

finely grated zest and juice of 1 unwaxed lemon, plus 1 more lemon, cut into wedges, to serve

4 sole fillets, skin on, each about 150g (5½oz)

watercress leaves

1 tablespoon chopped mint leaves

1 tablespoon chopped flat leaf parsley leaves

1 teaspoon red chilli flakes

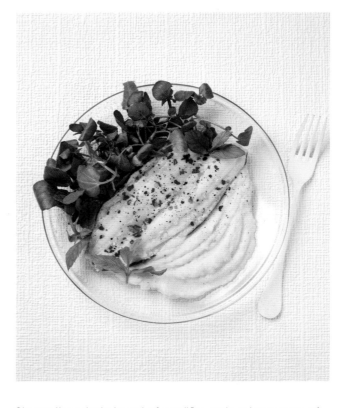

Steam the whole head of cauliflower in a large pan of boiling water until tender, about 8 minutes. Drain, break into florets, then blend with the cream and enough milk to reach your preferred consistency. Season to taste.

Meanwhile, preheat the grill to high and line a grill tray with foil. Melt the butter gently in a pan and add the lemon zest, juice and ½ teaspoon each of salt and black pepper. Now brush the top of the fish fillets with half the seasoned butter and grill, skin side up, for 5 minutes. Gently turn the fillets over and brush the other side with the remaining butter, grilling for a further 5 minutes, until tender.

Serve the sole on a bed of watercress, alongside the cauliflower cream. Garnish with lemon wedges and sprinkle with the chopped herbs and chilli flakes.

Sophie's Sausages & Smashing Beans

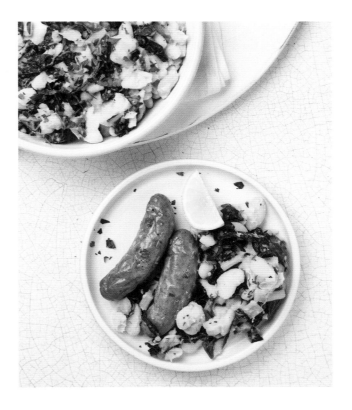

One of my favourite comfort food meals, this is hardly a recipe at all. Buy the best sausages you can afford, with the highest meat content. The lemony mash works beautifully with succulent pork sausages. Do vary the flavours of the smashed beans, by using garlic and spinach or even chilli and lime, if you like. For pork sausages, aim for less than 20% fat per 100g (3½oz), or, for an even leaner alternative, try chicken, venison or vegetarian sausages.

Serves 4

8 sausages

1 tablespoon good olive oil

200g (7oz) chard, sliced

½–1 garlic clove, crushed

1 teaspoon thyme leaves

2 × 400g (14oz) cans cannellini beans, drained and rinsed

400g (14oz) can butter beans, drained and rinsed

juice and zest of 1 lemon, plus extra to taste and lemon wedges to serve

sea salt and black pepper

good handful of chopped flat leaf parsley

Preheat the grill to medium.

Grill the sausages for 15–20 minutes, turning occasionally, until brown all over.

Meanwhile, in a shallow pan, heat the olive oil and fry the chard for 2 minutes, adding the garlic and thyme for the last 30 seconds. Set aside.

Add the beans to a pan and gently heat through over a medium heat. Remove from the heat and roughly smash the beans, lemon juice, salt and pepper together with a fork. Mix in the wilted chard and adjust the salt, lemon juice or pepper to taste.

Remove the sausages from the grill and drain on kitchen paper. Divide between plates with good dollops of the smashed beans.

Sprinkle with the parsley, add a little lemon zest and serve with a lemon wedge on the side.

Whole Roasted Sea Bass with Olives & Lemon

Serves 6

2–3 sea bass (roughly 400g/14oz each), heads off, scaled, gutted and cleaned

100ml (scant ½ cup) unsalted vegetable bouillon

100ml (scant ½ cup) dry white wine

zest of 1 unwaxed lemon, pared into strips with a veggie peeler

18 Kalamata olives

4–6 whole red peppercorns

½ teaspoon chilli flakes

good bunch of flat leaf parsley, chopped

sea salt

green vegetables, to serve

I love a 'bung in the oven and leave it' recipe and there are endless possibilities to baking a whole fish. I like this made with oily fish such as salmon, which works beautifully with the juice of an orange, white wine and orange zest. You can try adding capers and olives, for a Mediterranean nod – or ginger, lime and kaffir lime leaves for an Asian zing – into the cavity of any fish for extra flavour by slitting it open, stuffing and using toothpicks to hold the aromatics inside. Do play around... this is just one very simple version of baked fish.

Preheat the oven to 220°C/425°F/Gas Mark 7.

Place the fish whole in a roasting pan large enough for them to sit quite snugly.

Pour over the stock and wine and scatter the lemon zest, olives and peppercorns around the fish.

Roast in the oven until the flesh is tender, roughly 15 minutes, depending on the size of the fish.

Transfer to a serving dish and sprinkle with the chilli flakes, parsley and sea salt to taste.

Serve alongside any green vegetables. I tend to stick to a mix of mangetout, tenderstem broccoli and sugarsnap peas, lightly cooked and then shocked in ice cold water to maintain the crunch The juices of the fish will warm the veggies up.

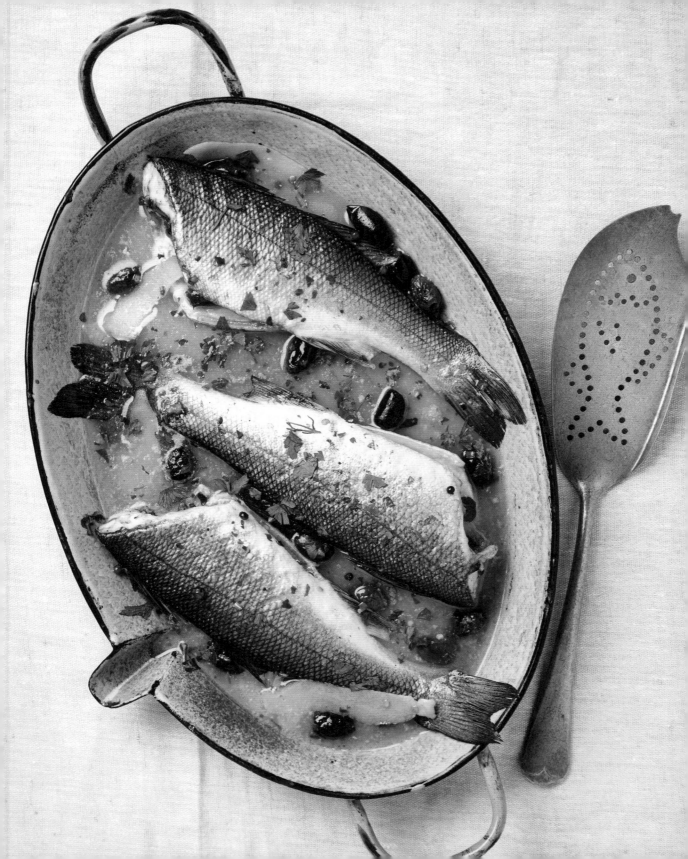

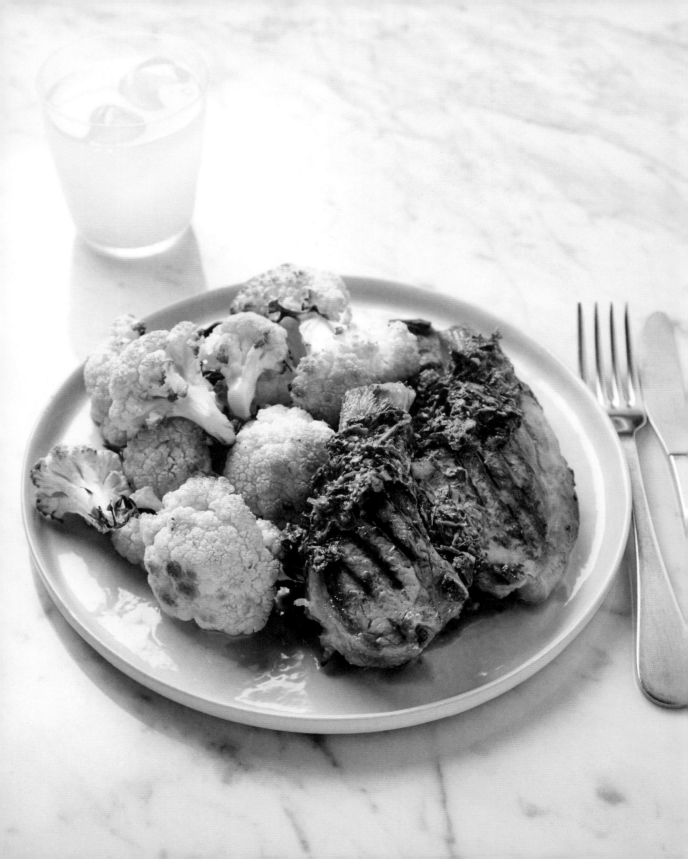

Lamb Cutlets with Salsa Verde

Serves 4

FOR THE CAULIFLOWER

1 cauliflower, cut into florets

1 tablespoon olive oil

1 garlic clove, finely chopped

leaves from 1 thyme sprig

FOR THE LAMB

4 x 200g (7oz) lamb cutlets
(allowing for bone)

1 tablespoon olive oil

1 garlic clove, halved

sea salt and black pepper

FOR THE SALSA VERDE

1 garlic clove

2 tablespoon capers

4 anchovy fillets

2 good handfuls of flat leaf
parsley leaves

1 tablespoon olive oil

1 tablespoon red wine vinegar

Salsa Verde gives you so much bang for your buck in terms of flavour, and will liven up any piece of fish or meat. Experiment with combinations until you find the right taste for you. Parsley is usually the foundation, but try adding basil or tarragon, cornichons, mustards and shallots.

Start with the cauliflower. Preheat the oven to 220°C/425°F/Gas Mark 7. Toss the cauliflower in the olive oil, garlic and thyme and roast for about 20 minutes, or until golden.

Meanwhile, prepare the lamb by brushing with olive oil and rubbing both sides of each cutlet with the garlic, and season well. Now griddle over a high heat for 3–4 minutes each side.

For the salsa verde, you can either use a pestle and mortar, knife or a mini blender. I prefer mine a little coarser and so I chop by hand; it retains a bright green colour and infuses the kitchen with the most wonderful aroma. Finely chop the garlic, capers, anchovies and parsley leaves. Combine with the olive oil, vinegar, salt and pepper and place in a small bowl to serve with the lamb and roasted cauliflower.

Milly's Appley Turkey Meatballs

Serves 8

FOR THE MEATBALLS

2 onions, grated

2 garlic cloves, grated

400g (1¾ cups) minced turkey

400g (1¾ cups) minced pork

2 apples, peeled and grated

handful of flat leaf parsley leaves, chopped

2 tablespoons grated Parmesan

2 eggs, lightly beaten

1½ teaspoons sea salt

½ teaspoon black pepper

3 tablespoons ground almonds

1 tablespoon light olive oil

FOR THE CHERRY TOMATO SAUCE

1 tablespoon olive oil

1 onion, grated

½ teaspoon dried parsley

1 garlic clove, grated

1 carrot, grated

400g (14oz) can cherry tomatoes

200g (1 cup) yellow cherry tomatoes, halved

These are super-simple to make and freeze well. They're a hit with kids and grown-ups alike, as they're sweet and gorgeously tender. Use turkey meat alone if you prefer but the pork does add tenderness. For a nut-free option use a slice of wholemeal bread instead of the ground almonds. Sometimes I make mini meatballs, thread them on to kebab sticks and reduce the sauce further to make a dipping sauce, somehow making the girls think I'm cooler than I am...

Preheat the oven to 220°C/425°F/Gas Mark 7.

Combine all the ingredients for the meatballs – except 2 tablespoons of the ground almonds and the oil – in a bowl (put the reserved almonds on a plate), and mix gently with a fork. You want the ingredients to be nicely combined, but don't overwork them or the meatballs will be tough.

Roll into 5cm (2 inch) balls and then roll in the remaining ground almonds until lightly coated. Heat the oil in a frying pan over a medium-high heat and cook the meatballs for 3–4 minutes, turning with a spoon, until a little browned. Now transfer to an baking tray lined with baking paper and bake for 20 minutes.

Meanwhile, prepare the tomato sauce. Heat the olive oil in the frying pan, adding the onion and stirring over a medium heat for 2 minutes. Now add the remaining ingredients and simply leave to simmer until the sauce is reduced and a little sticky, which will take 10–15 minutes.

You can either remove the baking paper from the baking tray, pour the sauce over the meatballs and bake in the oven for a further 5 minutes, or serve the meatballs with the sauce and extra green vegetables on the side.

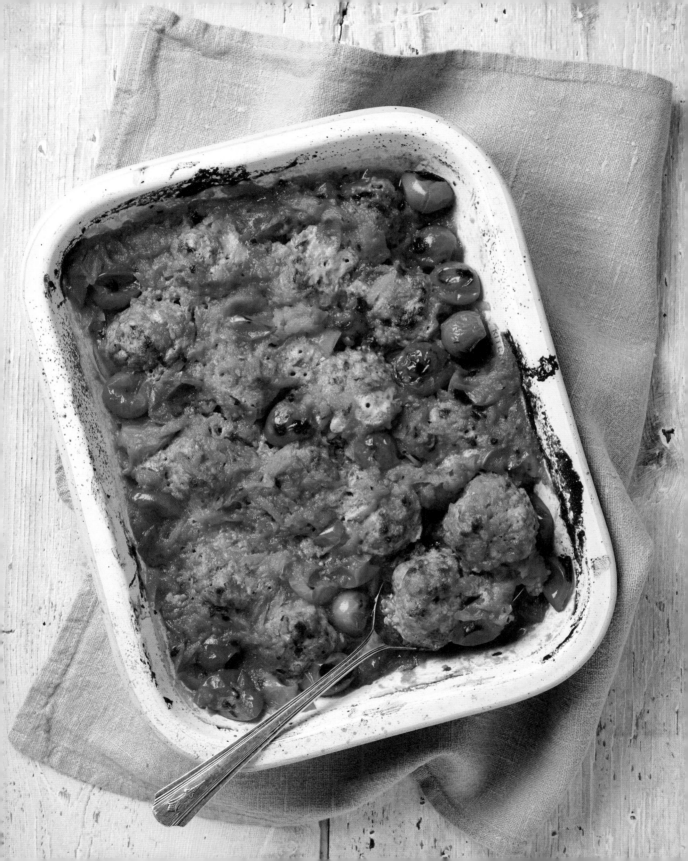

Our Nonna's Tray Bake

Serves 4

2 teaspoons sweet smoked paprika

1 tablespoon olive oil

2 red onions, quartered

2 yellow peppers, cut into chunks

100g (3½oz) Spanish Padron peppers, cut into chunks

100g (3½oz) chorizo, cut into chunks

2 garlic cloves, sliced

200g (7oz) fresh plum tomatoes

200g (7oz) green beans

1 tablespoon red wine vinegar

4 large skinless bone-in chicken thighs

good handful of flat leaf parsley, chopped, to serve

Nonna introduced me to this dish and it has turned into a total family favourite. I always serve it with the simplest of green salads, to cut through the rich flavours, but it's full of veg as it is, so you can also pop some spinach on the bottom of a shallow dish instead and portion the baked chicken and vegetables out in that, allowing the spinach to wilt underneath. Don't panic if you can't find the little Spanish Padron peppers... and be warned that about one in 10 are hot, so leave them out if you prefer less heat.

Preheat the oven to 200°C/400°F/Gas Mark 6.

Mix the sweet smoked paprika powder into the olive oil and spread evenly on a baking dish. Prepare the onions, peppers and Padron peppers and add to the baking dish, along with the chorizo and garlic.

Bake without the chicken for 20 minutes, giving it a gentle shake halfway through. Now add the tomatoes, green beans and vinegar and give it a gentle stir. Arrange the chicken on top and bake for a further 20 minutes in the centre of the oven. Sprinkle with plenty of flat leaf parsley to serve.

Serve with a simple green salad dressed with red wine vinegar.

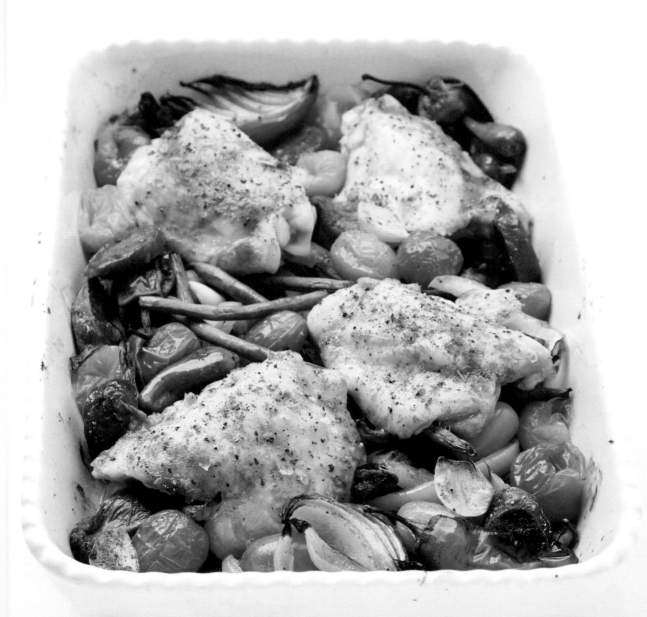

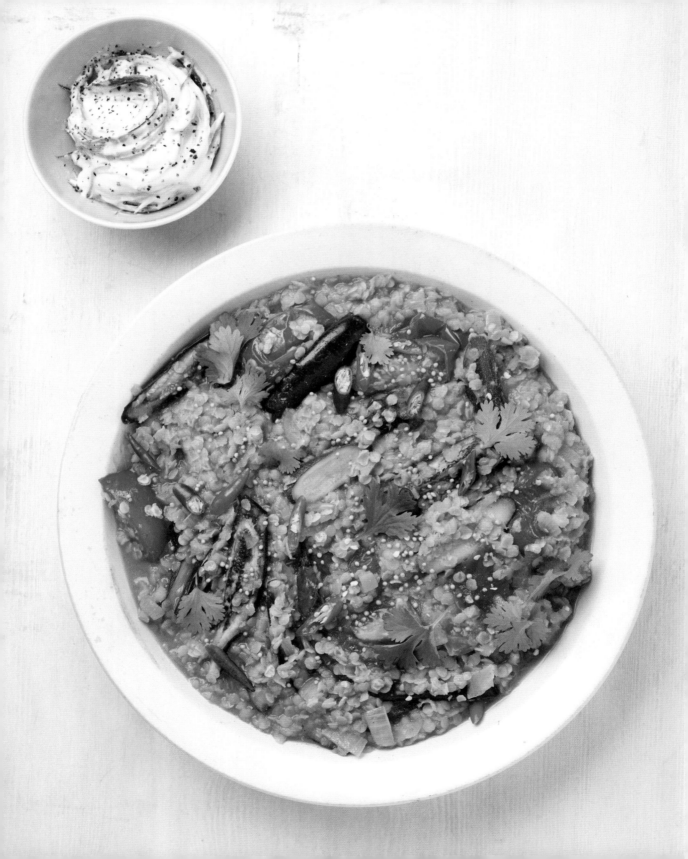

Grumpa's Creamy Courgette Dhal ⓥ

Serves 4

FOR THE DHAL

1½ tablespoons groundnut oil or ghee

4 onions, grated

1 tablespoon each ground cumin, ground coriander and curry powder

2 tablespoons (thumb-sized piece) peeled and grated fresh root ginger

8 tomatoes, roughly chopped

300g (1½ cups) chana dhal lentils, rinsed

1 whole garlic bulb, halved

4 green chillies, chopped, plus red or green chilli, to serve

4 carrots, grated

8 large courgettes, quartered

4 baby aubergines, halved

800ml (3¼ cups) vegetable stock

sea salt and black pepper

2 tablespoons mustard seeds

leaves from 1 bunch of coriander, roughly chopped

4 tablespoons coconut cream

FOR THE RAITA

½ cucumber, deseeded and chopped

300g (1¼ cups) 0% Greek yogurt

juice of 1 lemon

sea salt and black pepper

Nothing pleases me more than curry night at my parents. Daddy's chana dhal is so delicious, you'll make it time and time again. His secret is to cook it a couple of days before and, if you have a vegetable patch, it's a fantastic way of using up the inevitable glut of courgettes in the summer months, throwing any leftovers in the freezer for warming winter suppers, or to liven up a simple grilled piece of firm fish. Perfect for feeding large crowds on a budget. The girls love my mild version, and dip in steaming mini wholemeal pitta crisps for a light snack.

Heat 1 tablespoon of the groundnut oil or ghee in a casserole dish over a medium-low heat, add the onions and stir until very soft (about 5 minutes). Now add the spices and ginger, reduce the heat to low and stir for 2 minutes until fragrant.

Add the tomatoes and lentils and stir together until the lentils are coated. Simply throw in all of the remaining ingredients up to the mustard seeds (leave these out for now) and simmer for 30–40 minutes until the lentils are soft and beautifully thick. Add a dash of water if you prefer a looser consistency, and give it a good stir every 5 minutes or so to prevent sticking.

Meanwhile, pour the remaining oil or ghee into a small frying pan and fry the mustard seeds, lid on or they'll jump all over the kitchen. Set aside.

Mix together all the ingredients for the raita.

Now fish out the garlic and transfer the dhal to bowls. Sprinkle each with the toasted mustard seeds, coriander leaves, chilli and a drizzle of coconut cream. Serve with the raita.

Cider & Mustard Pork

Serves 4

FOR THE PORK

1 teaspoon cornflour

1 teaspoon English mustard powder

sea salt and black pepper

4 trimmed pork loin medallions or chops, each 150–175g (5½–6oz)

2 tablespoons olive oil

8 shallots, finely sliced

50ml (scant ¼ cup) cider

2 tablespoons wholegrain mustard

1 garlic clove, very finely chopped or crushed

150ml (⅔ cup) single cream

handful of flat leaf parsley, chopped

FOR THE APPLE SAUCE

2 Granny Smith apples, peeled and roughly chopped

1 Braeburn apple, skin on, chopped

FOR THE SAUTÉED PEES AND LETTUCE

200g (1½ cups) frozen peas

4–6 Cos lettuces, finely sliced

dash of cider

This is my version of a French classic, which works beautifully with lean pork tenderloins. It's usually made with pork chops, which you can do, but trim off the fat before eating. I love the sweetness of the sautéed lettuce and peas with the stabby-sharp taste of the cider. You can bash the medallions between sheets of cling film, to tenderize them further. Do batch-cook the apple sauce, as it's a faff to do for just one meal. It freezes well and can be stirred into Bircher muesli with cinnamon, or thrown into vanilla smoothies.

Preheat the oven to 190°C/375°F/Gas Mark 5.

On a flat plate, mix together the cornflour, mustard powder and seasoning and coat the medallions or chops on both sides.

Heat half the oil in a large frying pan and sear each medallion for 3–4 minutes on each side, until brown. Place in the oven for 15–20 minutes.

Put the apples in a small ovenproof dish with a dash of water and a tiny pinch of salt and cook in the oven for the same time as the pork. Simply give them a stir once they're done.

While the pork and apples are in the oven, prepare the mustard sauce. Cook the shallots very gently in the remaining tablespoon of olive oil until they are soft and caramelized. Increase the heat and add the cider until it deglazes the pan. Reduce the heat and add the wholegrain mustard and garlic, season with pepper and finally add the cream.

Now prepare the veggies by simply throwing the frozen peas and lettuce in a wok, with a little glug of cider and in 3–4 minutes they will be ready. Season to taste.

Sprinkle the pork with parsley and serve with the veggies, with a tablespoon or so of the mustard sauce and a dollop of apple sauce.

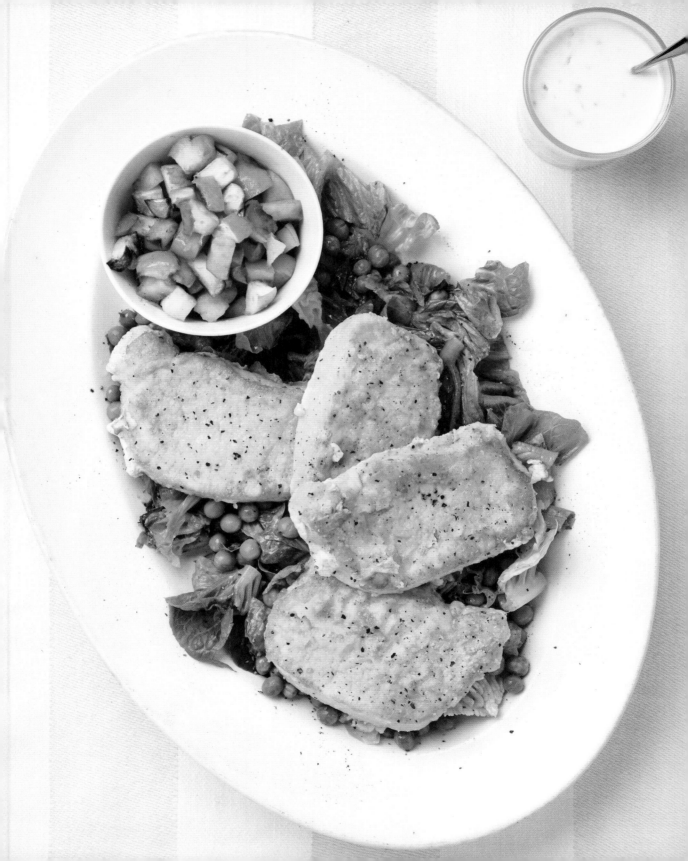

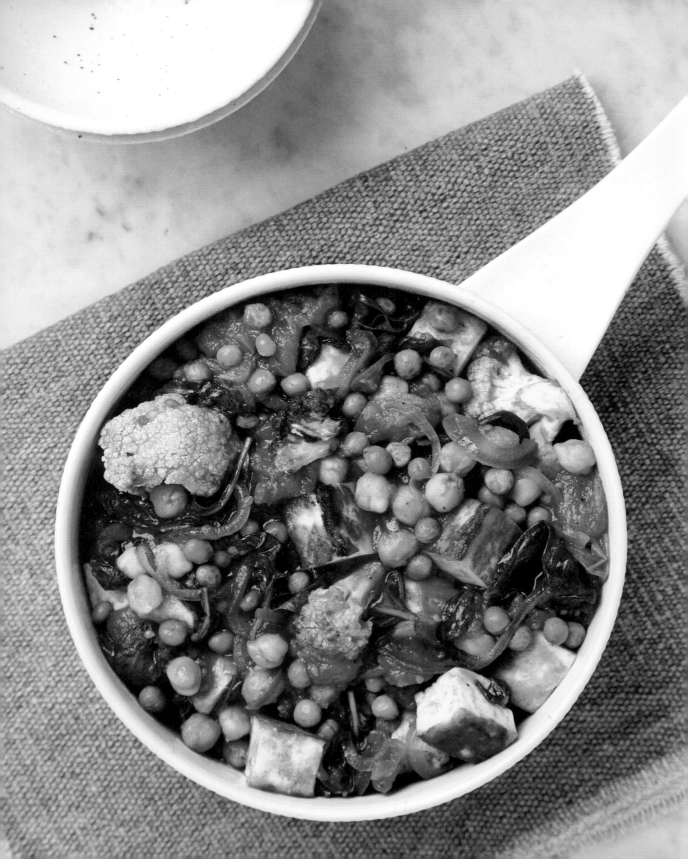

JP's Paneer & Cauliflower ⓥ

Serves 4

1 cauliflower

good spray of olive oil

8 garlic cloves, skin on

2 tablespoons groundnut oil

225g (8oz) pack of paneer cheese, cubed

2 red onions, finely sliced

1 teaspoon (1cm/½ inch piece) peeled and finely grated fresh root ginger

2 red chillies, chopped

¼ teaspoon garam masala

¼ teaspoon cayenne pepper

¼ teaspoon ground turmeric

2 x 400g (14oz) cans chopped or cherry tomatoes

400g (14oz) can chickpeas, drained and rinsed

200g (1½ cups) frozen peas

200g (7oz) frozen spinach, defrosted

sea salt and black pepper

leaves from 1 bunch of coriander, chopped

So deliciously simple that even my big brother can wow a crowd with this. It is relatively mild, so add more chillies if you fancy it. This is a wonderful vegetarian dish that tastes even better as leftovers, and I quite often serve it with leftover roast chicken. I use fresh spinach if I have it, but always keep frozen spinach and peas in my freezer. Don't shy away from frozen veg; they'll rescue you when the cupboards are bare and are arguably more nutritious than fresh. This makes a really cost-effective meal for a crowd.

Preheat the oven to 200°C/400°F/Gas Mark 6.

Chop the head of cauliflower into florets, spray lightly with olive oil and pop on a baking tray along with the garlic cloves. Bake for 20 minutes, until slightly golden. Remove and set aside.

Add 1 tablespoon of the groundnut oil to a wok and set over a medium heat. Brown the paneer cubes on all sides for about 5 minutes, then remove from the heat and set aside.

Add the remaining tablespoon of oil to the pan with the onions and keep stirring until they're golden. Add the ginger, chillies and ground spices and fry off the spices for 1 minute. Now add in the tomatoes and chickpeas, then squeeze the baked garlic from their skins into the pan and let it simmer over a low heat for 10–15 minutes. Add the paneer, cauliflower, peas and spinach and let the flavours combine and simmer over a very low heat for a further 5 minutes. Taste for seasoning and adjust to taste.

Sprinkle with plenty of coriander to serve.

Peppers with Four-hour Ragú & Garlic Cavolo Nero

Serves 8, and great for batch-cooking

FOR THE RAGÚ

1 tablespoon olive oil

2 large onions, finely chopped

50g (¼ cup) pancetta lardons

2 carrots, finely chopped

2 celery sticks, finely chopped

½ tablespoon dried oregano

½ tablespoon dried basil

400g (1¾ cups) lean minced pork

400g (1¾ cups) lean minced steak

2 x 400g (14oz) cans cherry tomatoes

½ beef jelly stock cube

250ml (1 cup) tomato passata

250ml (1 cup) good red wine

1 teaspoon black pepper

salt

leaves from a large bunch of basil

8 large red or yellow peppers

FOR THE CAVOLO NERO

1 tablespoon olive oil

2 garlic cloves, very finely sliced

400g (14oz) cavolo nero, finely sliced

This uses pork and is slow-cooked, resulting in the softest, richest ragú. You can serve it in peppers as I have done here, or on raw courgetti if you're not sick of it! My children also love it spread on toast for a quick midweek supper. Because we eat it so much, this recipe makes twice as much ragú as you need, so that you can freeze half.

Preheat the oven to 160°C/325°F/Gas Mark 3.

Heat the oil in a large ovenproof casserole dish over a medium heat and sweat the onions, pancetta, carrots and celery for 5 minutes. Add the dried herbs and stir for a further 5 minutes. Now add the minced pork and beef in little bits, breaking it up into little chunks with your wooden spoon until all the meat has browned. Stir in the cherry tomatoes including their juices, the stock cube, passata, wine and black pepper

Put the casserole in the oven, uncovered, for 4 hours, stirring every 30–45 minutes. Adjust the seasoning to taste and stir in all the basil.

Slice the stalk ends from the peppers (discard these) and scoop out and discard all the seeds. Stuff the peppers with the ragú, place on a baking tray and bake in the oven for 20–30 minutes, until the peppers are cooked but still firm.

When you're ready to eat, heat the 1 tablespoon of olive oil in a wok over a medium heat and add the garlic. Gently fry for 1 minute, taking care not to burn it, then add the cavolo nero, stirring and adding a splash of water every minute until it is softened and cooked, but still a little firm. Serve alongside the stuffed peppers.

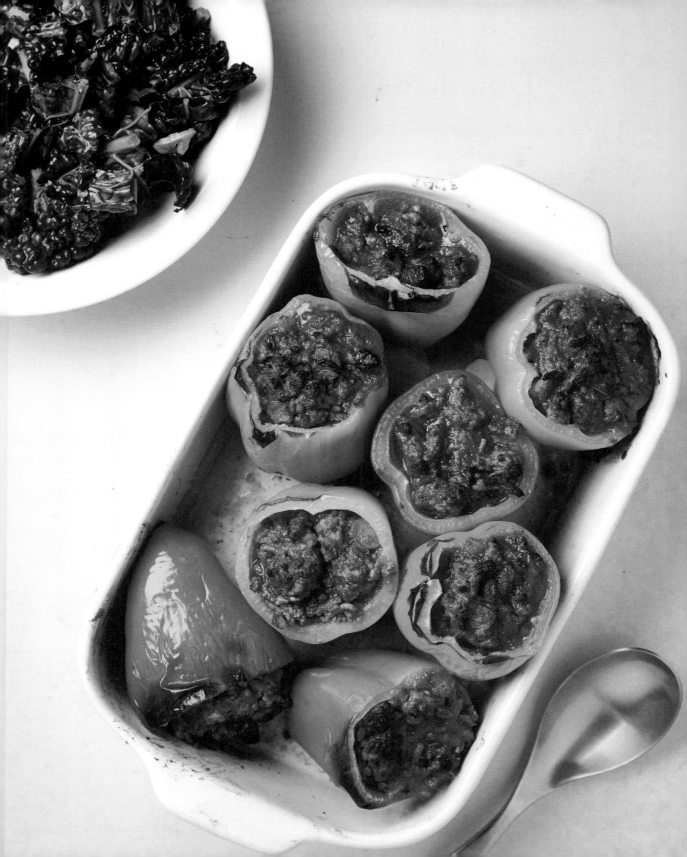

Double Bean Burger Balls ⓥ

Makes 8 large patties, or 20 mini balls
Your serving should be about 150g
(5½oz) of balls with a good tablespoon
of Avocado Hummus

FOR THE BEAN BURGER BALLS

1 slice of wholemeal bread

400g (14oz) can chickpeas,
drained and rinsed

400g (14oz) can butter beans,
drained and rinsed

1 teaspoon finely grated unwaxed
lemon zest

1 teaspoon ground cumin

1 tablespoon tahini

I garlic clove, peeled

1 teaspoon vegetable bouillion
powder

¼ teaspoon black pepper

1 large egg

handful of coriander, chopped

1 carrot, finely grated

1 large onion, grated

50g (⅓ cup) sunflower seeds

50g (½ cup) oatbran

1 tablespoon olive oil

Cos lettuce leaves, to serve

cherry tomatoes, to serve

Avocado Hummus, to serve
(see opposite)

This will make eight regular-sized patties, but I often roll them into mini balls that can be thrown on a salad or in a lunchbox. Don't be put off by the long ingredients list, as they're honestly super-quick to make. Spear mini balls on to little kebab sticks, adding tomatoes if you like, and dip them in my easy avocado hummus with a good side salad, then simply add a wholemeal bun or wrap for the kids. Try swapping the avocado for a roasted red pepper and some chilli for a lighter but equally delicious version.

Pop the slice of bread into the food processor and blitz for 20 seconds to make crumbs. Transfer to a large bowl. Now put the chickpeas and butter beans into the processor with the lemon zest, cumin, tahini, garlic, bouillion powder, pepper and the egg and blend until just combined. Scrape into the bowl of breadcrumbs and mix well with a fork, adding the coriander, grated carrot and onion, sunflower seeds and oatbran until you have a good moist mixture. Let stand for 10 minutes or until firm.

With clean hands, form into 8 large or 20 mini balls. Place on a plate and put in the fridge for 10 minutes before cooking.

Preheat the oven to 240°C/475°F/Gas Mark 9.

Brush the balls with olive oil and place on a baking tray lined with baking paper. Cook in the oven until nicely browned, 15–20 minutes.

Serve with crisp Cos lettuce, cherry tomatoes and avocado hummus (see opposite).

Avocado Hummus (Vg)

Makes 800g (3 cups)

400g (14oz) can chickpeas, drained and rinsed (keep a few back for decoration)

400g (14oz) can butter beans, drained and rinsed

2 tablespoons tahini

½ ripe avocado

1 garlic clove

1 lemon

sea salt

drizzle of olive oil

pinch of paprika

a little flat leaf parsley

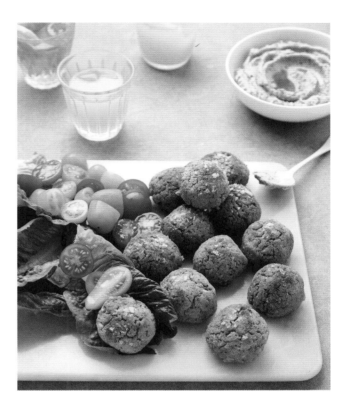

Add all the ingredients except the lemon, salt, olive oil, paprika and parsley to a food processor and pulse until really smooth. If you've the time, peel the skins off the butter beans and chickpeas first, for the creamiest hummus ever... I have to admit I don't have the patience for it, but it's a good job to give the kids while you're preparing dinner and chatting away.

Adjust the hummus to a consistency that suits you by adding more or less lemon juice and season to your own taste, though this takes a good bit of seasoning. Decorate with a drizzle of olive oil, some chickpeas, a pinch of paprika and some parsley. A good heaped tablespoon will provide you with protein to accompany the double bean burger balls (see opposite).

Ratatouille with Baked Eggs & Goats' Cheese ⓥ

Serves 4, plus another portion or so of ratatouille for the freezer

4 tablespoons olive oil

4 red onions, sliced

1 tablespoon herbes de Provençe

2 large aubergines, roughly chopped

2 red peppers, roughly chopped

2 yellow peppers, roughly chopped

700g (1lb 9oz) jar of tomato passata

2 x 400g (14oz) cans cherry tomatoes

1 garlic bulb, halved horizontally, skin on

black pepper

8 large courgettes, chunkily sliced

4 large eggs

200g (7oz) goats' cheese

good handful of basil leaves, to garnish

My ratatouille is a great way to use up slightly depressed veggies in the bottom drawer, combining them with a few kitchen cupboard basics. It's also very little effort and great for batch-cooking and keeping in the freezer. Serve with any leftover meats or fish or – as I love to do, as shown in this recipe – with baked eggs and chunks of creamy goats' cheese.

Preheat the oven to 200°C/400°F/Gas Mark 6.

In a large ovenproof pan, over a low heat, heat the olive oil. Add the red onions and keep stirring for 10 minutes until they are soft and begin to caramelize. Add the dried herbs and increase the heat to medium.

Add the aubergines, peppers, passata and tomatoes and stir, then tuck in the garlic and season with black pepper to taste.

Bring to a simmer, then transfer to the oven, lid off, and cook for 20 minutes. Now add the courgettes and cook for a further 10 minutes. Allow to cool. Now is the time to store the ratatouille you won't need in handy portion sizes in freezer bags, if you want to.

To serve 4, transfer 6 soup ladles of the ratatouille to a baking dish and make 4 hollows in the top. Break an egg into each hollow, sprinkle with chunks of goats' cheese and bake in the oven until the eggs are cooked through and the cheese melts into the dish. Garnish with basil.

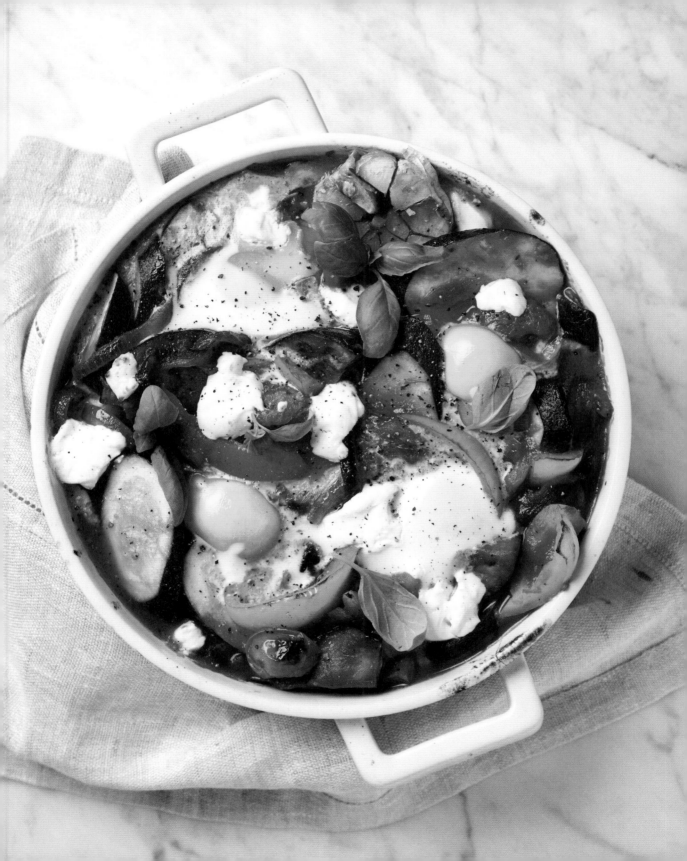

Catania Cod Tray Bake

I love tray bakes – they are a really simple way to intensify flavours... and minimize preparation and washing-up at the same time! Do play around and mix up the ingredients; it's all about experimenting. This works well with all firm white fish, and is wonderful with chicken thighs, too.

Serves 4

2 red onions

250g (9oz) yellow cherry tomatoes, on the vine

250g (9oz) red cherry tomatoes, on the vine

8 caperberries

2 thyme sprigs

juice and finely grated zest of 1 unwaxed lemon

1 garlic clove, sliced

1 tablespoon olive oil

sea salt and black pepper

8 large green olives, pitted and sliced

300g (10½oz) tenderstem broccoli

1 teaspoon green pesto

4 x 125g (4½oz) cod fillets

4 large slices of prosciutto

good handful of chopped flat leaf parsley

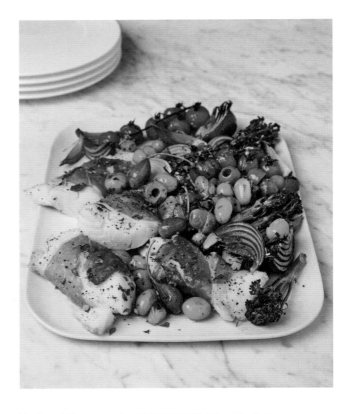

Preheat the oven to 220°C/425°F/Gas Mark 7.

Cut the onion into eighths (don't chop the ends off as this holds the chunks together nicely) and arrange on a large baking tray, ideally one with shallow sides to avoid the vegetables steaming, we want them to crisp up. Add the cherry tomatoes, caperberries, thyme, lemon zest, garlic and olive oil. Add salt and pepper and roast for 15 minutes. After 15 minutes, add the sliced olives, broccoli and pesto and very gently stir the contents of the baking tray.

Wrap each cod fillet in a slice of prosciutto, make a space in the centre of the baking tray and place the cod there. Roast for a further 15 minutes or until the cod is golden, but still delicately white in the centre.

Remove from the oven, squeezing the lemon juice over the tray. Serve with plenty of chopped parsley.

Toff's Niçoise

This salad is basically a simple assembly job and can easily be simplified even further by using 4 large eggs instead of the quails' eggs. Do leave out the lumpfish caviar if you prefer, although it adds a bit of pomp for a couple of quid, if that.

Serves 4

200g (7oz) French beans

400g (14oz) baby leaf salad

20 large green olives, sliced

4 tablespoons capers

1 red onion, finely sliced

4 x 125g (4½oz) poached salmon fillets

12 quails' eggs, soft boiled, peeled and halved

8 fresh anchovy fillets

2–4 teaspoons lumpfish caviar, to taste

handful of dill, finely chopped

1 quantity Classic French Dressing (see page 122)

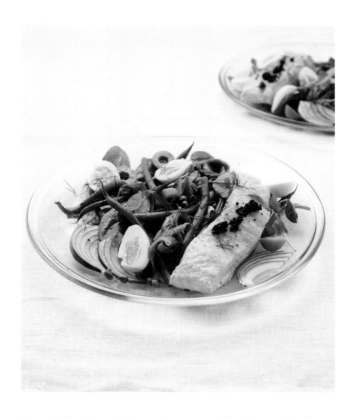

Blanch the French beans in a pan of boiling water for 4–5 minutes, then transfer immediately to a large bowl of cold water and ice cubes for 2 minutes to stop the cooking. Drain.

Arrange the base salad ingredients – French beans, salad leaves, olives, capers and red onion – on a large platter or individual serving plates.

Now place the salmon on top, scatter with the quails' eggs, drape with the anchovies and add a few dollops of caviar. Sprinkle evenly with the dill to finish.

Serve alongside a bowl of the French dressing for everyone to help themselves.

Turkey, Leek & Bacon Pie

Serves 8

FOR THE FILLING

150g (5½oz) pancetta lardons

4 large leeks, finely sliced

2 large carrots, chopped

2 celery stalks, chopped

2 garlic cloves, chopped

1 thyme sprig

1 tablespoon cornflour

small knob (pat) of unsalted butter

800g (1lb 12oz) cooked turkey meat

250ml (1 cup) good chicken stock, plus more if needed

sea salt and black pepper

200g (7oz) full-fat Greek yogurt

FOR THE TOPPING

2 parsnips, roughly chopped

1 cauliflower

1 vegetable bouillon cube

3½ tablespoons unsalted butter

50ml (scant ¼ cup) milk (optional)

50g (½ cup) grated Parmesan cheese

To cut through the richness of this dish, I like to serve it with a green salad, simply dressed in good white wine or champagne vinegar.

Firstly, prepare the filling. In a large saucepan, fry off the pancetta until browned, then remove, keeping the fat in the pan, and place the pancetta on kitchen paper to soak up the excess fat. Now, over a medium heat, gently sauté the leeks, carrots, celery, garlic and thyme in the pancetta fat.

Meanwhile, blend the cornflour into the butter until it is very smooth.

Add the turkey to the vegetables pan (in chunks or simply torn off the bird), then return the pancetta and sauté for just a minute or so until the flavours combine. Now add in the cornflour and stock, bit by bit, until the sauce thickens beautifully. Adjust the amount of stock until you reach your desired consistency and taste for seasoning. Add the Greek yogurt (low-fat may curdle, so do use full-fat Greek yogurt here).

Prepare the topping by steaming the parsnips and cauliflower, with the bouillon cube added to the water in the steamer for extra flavour. Remove and blend, along with the butter. You can add a little milk if you'd like a smoother consistency. Preheat the grill to high.

Transfer the filling to a pie dish, smother the top with the blended vegetables and sprinkle with the grated Parmesan.

Pop the pie under the grill, keeping a close eye on it, until a golden crust begins to form. Serve with extra green vegetables. I love it with gently sautééd spinach.

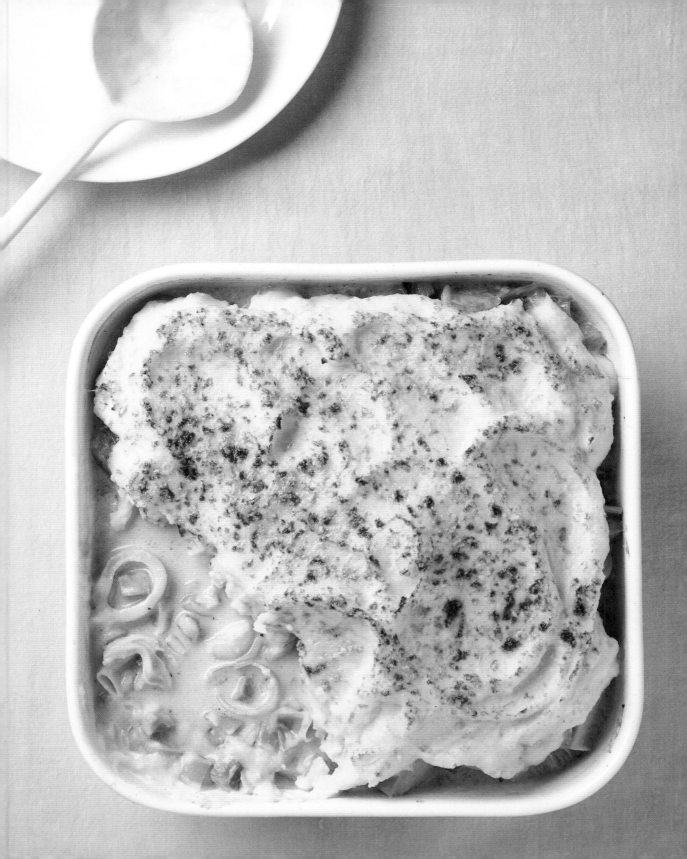

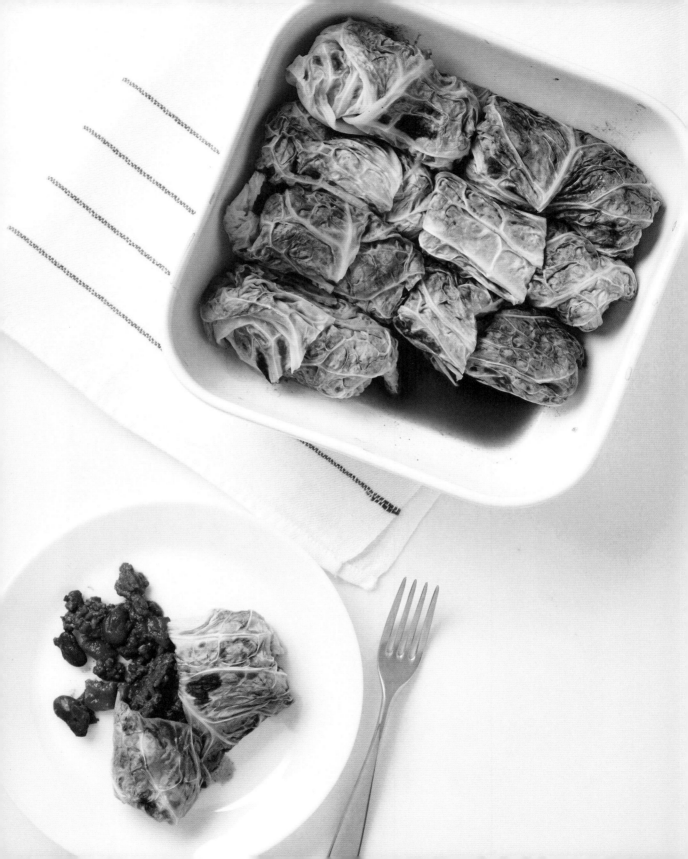

CoCo's Chocolate Con Carne Pressies

Serves 8 (a portion is 2–3 pressies per person)

1 tablespoon olive oil

2 onions, finely chopped

800g (3½ cups) lean minced steak, or Quorn mince

2 garlic cloves, very finely chopped or crushed

2 x 400g (14oz) cans cherry tomatoes

250ml (1 cup) water

2 teaspoons chilli powder

2 red peppers, chopped

½ beef jelly stock cube (or vegetable if you're using Quorn)

¾ teaspoon black pepper

2 tablespoons cocoa powder

400g (14oz) can red kidney beans, drained and rinsed (optional)

1 whole Savoy cabbage

I often batch-cook vast cauldrons of this and split it, about 30 minutes before it's ready, into two pots. I'll add in a huge bunch of mini peppers and chillies for the grown-ups, so I've two versions ready to defrost for a quick midweek supper. This works really well with Quorn, too, for a meat-free Monday. You can, of course, serve this with brown rice for the family on the side, but, for a lower-carb version, the little cabbage wraps work so well.

Preheat the oven to 160°C/325°F/Gas Mark 3.

Heat the oil in an ovenproof casserole dish and sweat the onions over a medium-low heat until transparent, about 3 minutes. Add the minced meat and stir for a further 5 minutes until nicely browned, breaking up the chunks as you go. Now add the garlic, tomatoes, water, chilli powder, red peppers, stock cube, black pepper, cocoa powder and kidney beans, if using, and give it all a quick stir. Transfer to the oven, uncovered, and cook slowly for 1½ hours, giving it a stir every 30 minutes or so.

Meanwhile, immerse the whole cabbage in a large pan of boiling water and simmer for 4–5 minutes, until the leaves are a little softened. Remove and wait for it to cool. Peel off the leaves, using only those that are firm enough to hold the filling.

Now make the pressies. Take 1 leaf at a time and trim off the coarse stem. The leaf should be facing upward (the side that was inside the cabbage should be facing you), in a bowl shape. Take 2 tablespoons of the meat mixture and place it on the leaf. Bring the bottom of the leaf up and over the filling and then fold the right edge of the leaf inward. Leave the left side open. Continue rolling the leaf from the bottom up, then tuck the loose end into the centre of the pressie.

Increase the oven temperature to 190°C/375°F/Gas Mark 5. Return the parcels to the oven for 20 minutes.

6

FAST FIT FOOD

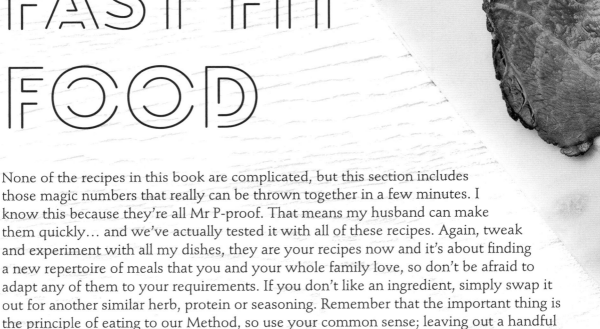

None of the recipes in this book are complicated, but this section includes those magic numbers that really can be thrown together in a few minutes. I know this because they're all Mr P-proof. That means my husband can make them quickly… and we've actually tested it with all of these recipes. Again, tweak and experiment with all my dishes, they are your recipes now and it's about finding a new repertoire of meals that you and your whole family love, so don't be afraid to adapt any of them to your requirements. If you don't like an ingredient, simply swap it out for another similar herb, protein or seasoning. Remember that the important thing is the principle of eating to our Method, so use your common sense; leaving out a handful of coriander won't affect your results. Eating a double portion will.

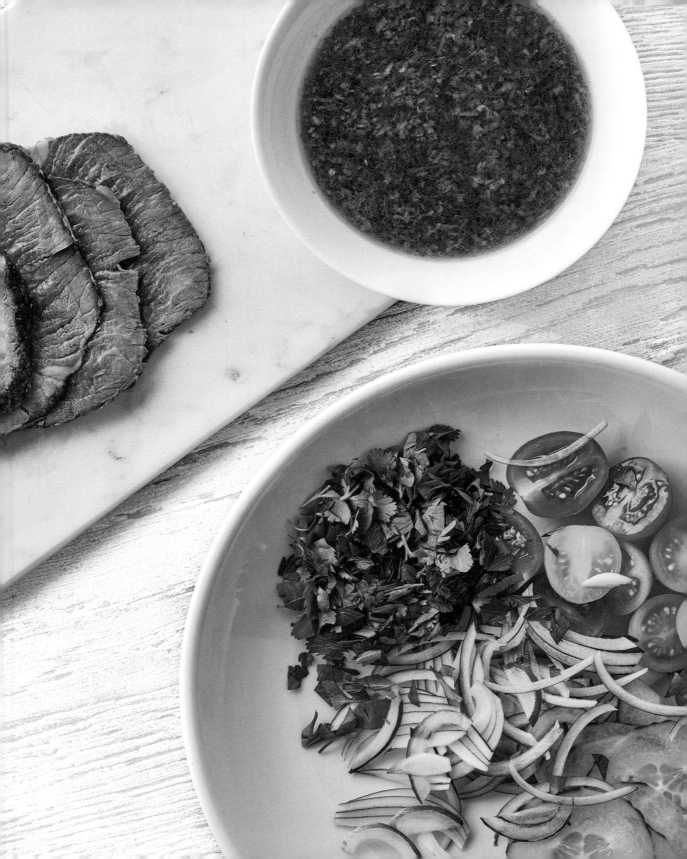

Salmon with 2-minute Pesto

This is ridiculously easy and rich, so it does need the balance of the very lemony kale to cut through the topping. You can vary the topping with all sorts of herbs, seeds and zests and – once you're in the Lifestyle phase – swap the bread for Japanese panko crumbs, which will give you a much crunchier topping.

Serves 4

FOR THE SALMON

4 x 17(6oz) salmon fillets

juice of 1 lemon, plus lemon wedges, to serve

½ slice of wholemeal bread

1 tablespoon pine nuts

1 tablespoon walnuts

2 tablespoons grated pecorino cheese

good handful of basil

½ teaspoon black pepper

½ teaspoon sea salt

FOR THE KALE

1 tablespoon olive oil

500g (1lb 2oz) curly kale, coarse stems discarded, torn into bite-sized pieces

juice of 1 lemon

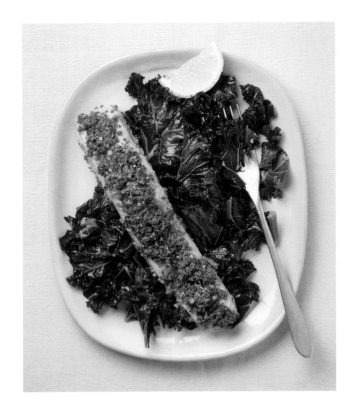

Preheat the oven to 240°C/475°F/Gas Mark 9.

Place the salmon fillets on a baking tray, give them a good squeeze of lemon juice and set aside.

Blitz all the remaining ingredients in a mini-blender for 30 seconds, until well mixed but a little chunky.

Divide the topping evenly over the salmon and place in the middle of the oven for 10–12 minutes. The topping should be beautifully crisp and the inside a little rare.

Meanwhile, for the kale, heat the olive oil in a large wok over a medium heat, adding the kale bit by bit until it reduces and cooks down. Keep adding a splash of water to steam-fry every minute or so, and keep stirring. I like it relatively well cooked, but go with your preference; mine takes 6–8 minutes. Drench in lemon juice and season very well.

Remove the salmon from the oven and serve alongside the kale, with lemon wedges.

Bubble & Squeak

I use pancetta here, but this recipe is gorgeous too with ham hock or chorizo or – if you're veggie – leave out the bacon completely and you won't be disappointed. And, of course, the sprouts are optional; swap in Savoy cabbage if you prefer. I always cook extra veg, always al dente, so that it's ready to bolster a salad or turn into this ultimate leftover meal.

Serves 4

75g (¾ cup) pancetta lardons

2 red onions, finely chopped

4 carrots, finely chopped

2 celery sticks, finely chopped

150g (1½ cups) Brussels sprouts, shredded

150g (1 cup) peas

1 garlic clove, very finely chopped or crushed

400g (4 cups) chard, shredded

1 tablespoon Worcestershire sauce

sea salt and black pepper

4 large eggs

good handful of chopped flat leaf parsley leaves

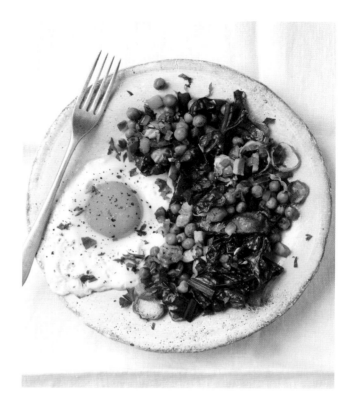

Throw the pancetta straight into a frying pan or wok, over a medium heat, with the onions, carrots and celery and fry for 2 minutes. Now increase the heat, add the sprouts and peas and keep stirring until everything begins to turn a little crunchy.

Reduce the heat and add the garlic and chard, adjusting the heat to avoid burning (which will impart an acrid taste). Splash in the Worcestershire sauce and give it a good stir for a minute. Taste and season accordingly and set aside.

Fry or poach the eggs and serve on top of each portion of bubble and squeak, sprinkling well with parsley.

Mini Chicken Parmesan

Serves 4

FOR THE CHICKEN

1 slice of wholemeal bread, crumbed

2 tablespoons oatbran

1 teaspoon dried sage

1 teaspoon dried thyme

1 teaspoon dried oregano

4 tablespoons finely grated Parmesan

1 tablespoon English mustard powder

sea salt and black pepper

2 large eggs

600g (1lb 5oz) mini chicken fillets

1 tablespoon olive oil

FOR THE SALAD

2 green apples

½ cucumber, deseeded

100g (3½oz) sugarsnap peas

juice of 1 lemon

200g (8 packed cups) baby spinach

200g (8 packed cups) wild rocket

2 tablespoons Classic French Dressing
(see page 122)

For an even crunchier coating you can bake the oatmeal mixture in the oven for 5 minutes before using it to coat the chicken, but I find it is crispy enough anyway as it is.

Preheat the oven to 200°C/400°F/Gas Mark 6.

In a bowl, mix the breadcrumbs, oatbran, dried herbs, Parmesan, mustard power and salt and pepper. Beat the eggs well and put into a shallow dish. Dip the chicken into the eggs all over, before coating well in the dry mixture.

Brush a baking tray with the olive oil, transfer the chicken to the tray and bake in the centre of the oven for 12 minutes

Prepare the salad by slicing the apples, cucumber and sugarsnap peas into fine sticks and drenching in the lemon juice to prevent the apples from browning. Combine in a bowl with the spinach and rocket. Toss the salad with the dressing and serve the chicken fillets on top. Or you can also chop the fillets when piping hot and stir into the salad, which is lovely in winter as the spinach and rocket warms and wilts a little.

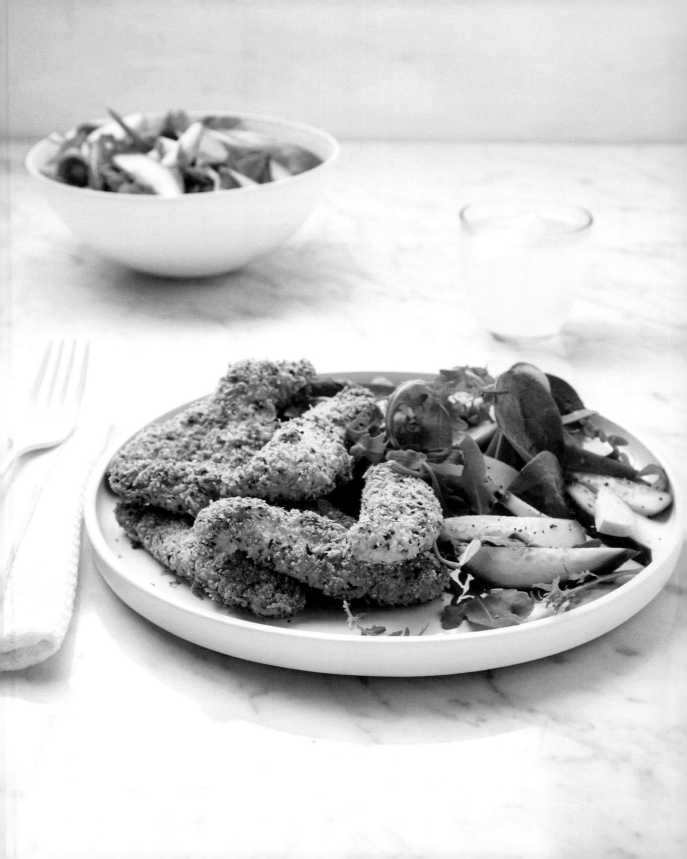

Ten-minute Thai Beef Salad

Serves 4

FOR THE SALAD

1 cucumber, sliced

400g (2 cups) cherry tomatoes, halved

1 red onion, halved and finely sliced

leaves from 1 bunch of coriander, roughly chopped, plus a few extra leaves to serve

leaves from 1 bunch of flat leaf parsley, roughly chopped

leaves from 1 bunch of Thai basil, roughly chopped, plus a few large leaves to serve

600-800g (1lb 5oz–1lb 12oz) leftover roast beef, or cooked steak, sliced

2 tablespoons chopped toasted peanuts

FOR THE DRESSING

2 tablespoons sesame oil

juice of 2 limes

1 tablespoon fish sauce

2 garlic cloves, very finely chopped or crushed

zest of ½ unwaxed lime

1 teaspoon (1cm/½ inch piece) peeled and very finely chopped or grated fresh root ginger

¼–½ teaspoon stevia, to taste

2 teaspoons reduced-sodium soy sauce

1–2 red chillies, very finely chopped, to taste

This is a great way to use up Sunday's leftover roast beef... and takes me back to balmy nights on the beach in Koh Phi Phi – from a dreary Monday night in my kitchen – in no time at all. If you haven't got any leftover beef, fry up a couple of bavette steaks, which are really good value and seriously full of flavour. You eat with your eyes so you can use a mixture of red, green and yellow tomatoes to make this salad even prettier. Don't assume the kids won't love it either; add the chilli only to the plates that want it just before serving.

Assemble all the ingredients for the salad – except the beef and peanuts – on a large, flat platter.

Now make the dressing, by simply whisking the ingredients together until the stevia has dissolved. Do taste and add more chilli if you like more heat, or more stevia if you like a bit more sweetness.

Arrange the beef in slices on top of the salad and dress the platter evenly with the dressing. Garnish with warm, toasted peanuts and more Thai basil to serve.

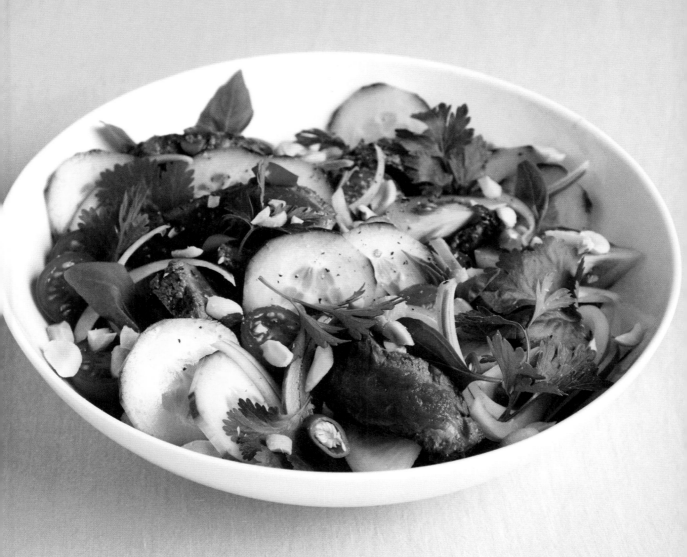

FRITTATA 4 WAYS

Fritattas are filling, versatile and a great way to use up leftovers. They're fabulous cold, so make extra to have leftovers for work. They'll keep well for a couple of days in the fridge.

You can also cook these in sheet pans, then cut them up into little squares and pop them on skewers, so that the kids will love them too.

① Basic Frittata Ⓥ

Serves 4

1 tablespoon olive oil

1 red onion, finely chopped

½ carrot, finely chopped

8 large eggs

sea salt and black pepper

Preheat the grill to medium. Heat the oil in a large omelette pan over a medium heat and fry the onion and carrot until lightly cooked.

Beat the eggs really well and season with salt and pepper. Add the eggs to the pan and cook over a medium heat for 5 minutes until the sides begin to set.

Now pop under the grill for 5 minutes, keeping an eye on it, until the top has just set.

② Goats' Cheese & Tomato Ⓥ

Serves 4

1 tablespoon olive oil

1 red onion, finely chopped

½ carrot, finely chopped

½ celery stick, finely chopped

handful of fresh thyme, chopped

200g (1 cup) each red and yellow cherry tomatoes

8 large eggs

sea salt and black pepper

handful of basil leaves, sliced

150g (1 cup) goats' cheese, crumbled or sliced

Preheat the grill to medium. Heat the oil in a large omelette pan over a medium heat and fry the onion, carrot, celery and thyme until lightly cooked.

Now add the tomatoes and fry gently until they become gooey and the liquid has cooked off.

Beat the eggs really well and season with salt and pepper. Add the eggs and basil to the pan and cook for 5 minutes until the sides begin to set.

Scatter the top with goats' cheese and pop under the grill for 5 minutes, keeping an eye on it, until the top has set and the cheese begins to turn golden.

③ Marsala Onions, Chorizo & Manchego

Serves 4

1 tablespoon olive oil

knob (pat) of unsalted butter

4 large white onions, finely sliced

1 tablespoon Marsala wine

100g (⅓ cup) chorizo, finely chopped

8 large eggs

sea salt and black pepper

handful of chopped flat leaf parsley leaves

50g (½ cup) Manchego cheese, grated

Heat the oil and butter in a large omelette pan over a medium-low heat and fry the onions slowly and gently for 10 minutes, until they become super-soft, brown and caramelized.

Preheat the grill to medium.

Add the Marsala wine to deglaze the pan, stirring to remove all the delicious brown bits. The onions should be soft, sticky and not crispy. Set aside in a bowl.

Now fry the chorizo in the same pan, until it begins to crisp. Beat the eggs really well and season with salt and pepper. Add the eggs, onions and parsley to the pan and give them a gentle twirl.

Cook over a medium heat for 5 minutes until the sides begin to set. Scatter with the Manchego and pop under the grill for 5 minutes, keeping an eye on it, until the top has set and the cheese begins to turn golden.

④ Leek, Ham & Petits Pois

Serves 4

1 tablespoon olive oil

2 leeks, finely sliced

½ carrot, finely chopped

½ celery stick, finely chopped

½ teaspoon dried thyme

200g (1½ cups) frozen petits pois

8 large eggs

sea salt and black pepper

90g (¼ cup) cooked ham hock, chopped

handful of mint leaves, chopped

50g (½ cup) pecorino or Parmesan, finely grated

Preheat the grill to medium. Heat the oil in a large omelette pan over a medium heat and fry the leeks, carrot, celery and dried thyme until lightly cooked.

Now add the frozen peas and fry gently until they defrost and combine with the veggies.

Beat the eggs really well and season with salt and pepper. Add the eggs, ham and mint to the pan and cook over a medium heat for 5 minutes until the sides begin to set.

Scatter the top of the frittata with the pecorino or Parmesan and pop under the grill for 5 minutes, keeping an eye on it, until the top has set and the cheese begins to turn golden.

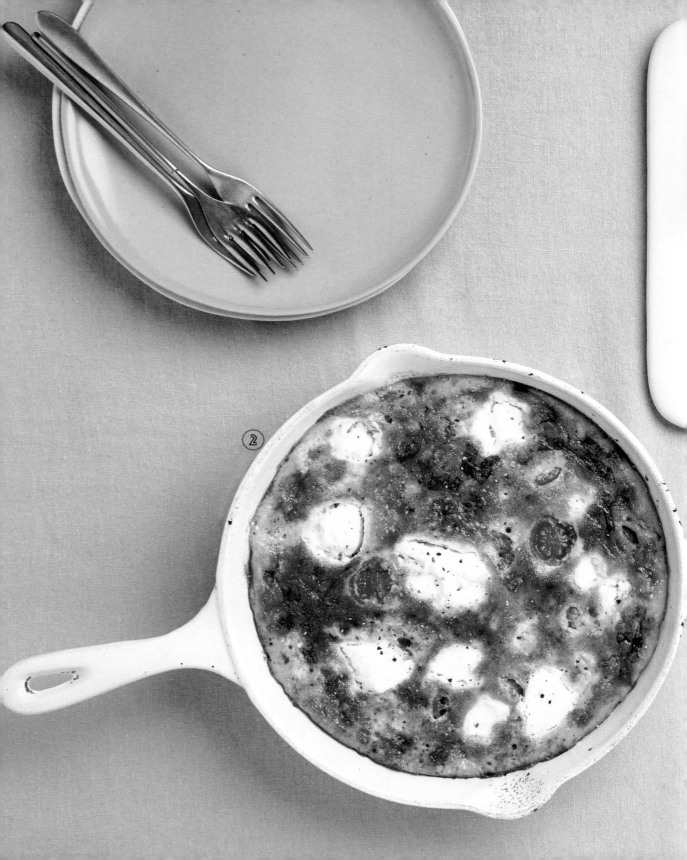

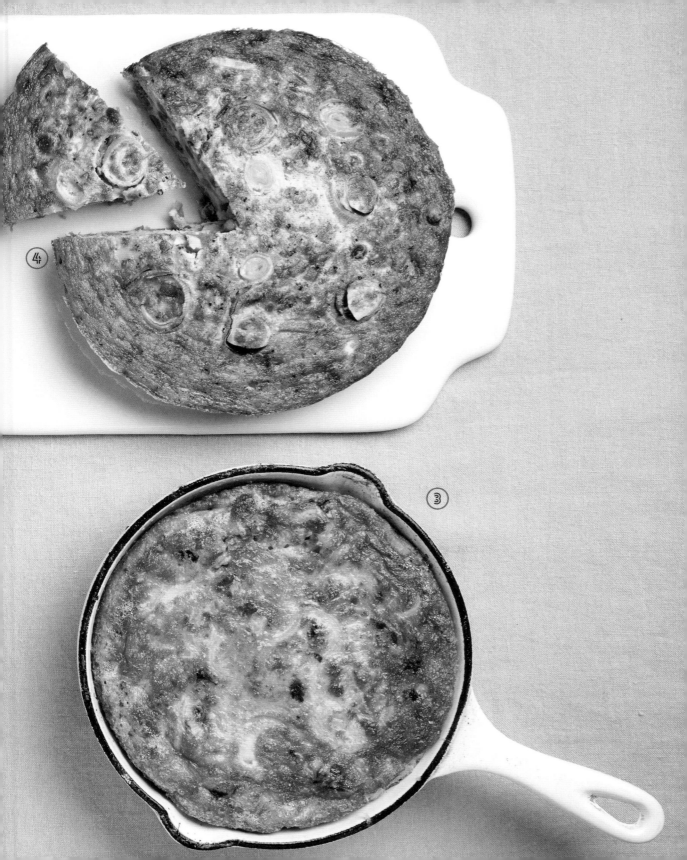

Black Pepper Stir-Fry

This is one of my favourite suppers. Adding the tomatoes at the end gives a lovely sweetness to balance the black pepper, and with so many vegetables you won't miss rice or noodles at all. Be sure not to skip any of the finishing touches, they make all the difference.

Serves 4

4 teaspoons black peppercorns

2 tablespoons sesame oil

2 tablespoons groundnut oil

600g (1lb 5oz) tiger prawns

8 spring onions, cut into thirds

4 medium-hot red chillies, to taste

2 teaspoons fish sauce

2 teaspoons finely grated fresh root ginger

2 teaspoons finely grated garlic

1 head of broccoli, cut into florets

4 red peppers, sliced

200g (7oz) mangetout, cut into strips

2 tablespoons reduced-sodium soy sauce

300g (1½ cups) cherry tomatoes

TO FINISH

good bunch of coriander, chopped

2 spring onions, sliced

2 red chillies, finely sliced

juice of 3 limes

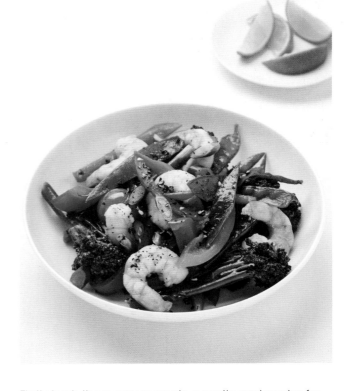

Firstly bash the peppercorns in a pestle and mortar for the best flavour. Add half the sesame oil and groundnut oil to a hot wok and stir-fry the prawns, spring onions, chillies and fish sauce for a couple of minutes, before adding the ginger and garlic. Now add the cracked black pepper and cook for a further minute. Remove from the pan and set aside.

In the same wok, use the remaining sesame and groundnut oils to stir-fry the vegetables except the tomatoes for 2 minutes over a high heat. Add a dash of water and soy sauce to deglaze the pan and help the veggies to steam-fry a little. Now add the tomatoes and stir-fry until they begin to pop. Return the prawns.

Working quickly, remove the stir-fry from the heat and finish with the coriander, spring onions and chillies, then dress with the juice of the limes. Serve immediately.

Paul's Passion Fruit Chicken

I've never seen my husband quite as proud as he was the night he accidently invented this dish. Poor bloke was home alone, with nothing but chicken fillets, wrinkly passion fruits and a Cos lettuce in the fridge. I'm loathe to admit it, but it's damn good and I love it for a light supper when I fancy something zingy, fresh and idiot-proof.

Serves 4

FOR THE CHICKEN

1 tablespoon olive oil

1 tablespoon jerk seasoning

4 x 150g (5½oz) mini chicken fillets

whole Little Gem leaves, to serve

FOR THE DRESSING

1 tablespoon olive oil

pulp of 4 passion fruit

juice of 2 limes

sea salt and black pepper

pinch of stevia

FOR THE SALSA

2 handfuls coriander, chopped

4 spring onions, finely chopped

2 red chillies, finely chopped

4 tomatoes, deseeded and chopped

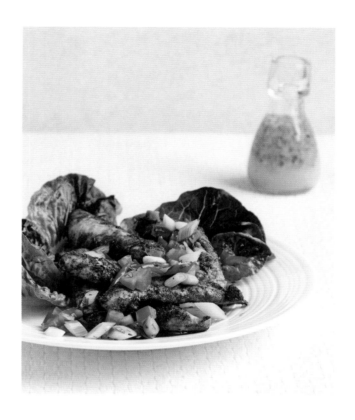

Preheat the oven to 200°C/400°F/Gas Mark 6.

Blend together the olive oil and jerk seasoning and use this to marinate the chicken, coating it thoroughly, ideally for 1 hour (but I quite often rush it in 5 minutes). Place on a baking tray and cook for 10–12 minutes until cooked through. Set aside to cool.

Meanwhile, prepare the dressing by simply whisking together all the ingredients. Add the stevia last, and only if you fancy a little extra sweetness, as this will depend on how ripe your fruit is. Add it slowly, as too much can ruin it and you can't take it out.

Now mix together all the ingredients for the salsa.

You can either tear up the chicken fillets into little shreds, or just place them whole into little crispy lettuce leaves, top with some salsa and a little dressing. Get messy and enjoy.

Salmon & Artichoke Tray Bake

Serves 4

FOR THE TRAY BAKE

a little olive oil

400g (14oz) jarred artichoke hearts in oil (drained weight)

400g (14oz) asparagus spears

4 x 150g (5½oz) salmon fillets

100ml (scant ½ cup) dry white wine

sea salt and black pepper

1 lemon or orange, plus lemon or orange wedges, to serve

handful of dill, chopped

FOR THE TOPPING

2 tablespoons flaked almonds

1 tablespoon pesto

½ teaspoon finely grated unwaxed lemon zest

Fresh artichokes are one of my favourite foods and I loved eating my dad's home-grown ones with him as a child... I think partly because they allowed so much time sitting on his lap, peeling away the leaves and learning to carve out the heart like a surgeon. As lovely as they are when fresh, they're a faff, so I cheat and use ready-prepared hearts in olive oil, which work brilliantly in this tray bake.

Preheat the oven to 220°C/425°F/Gas Mark 7.

Lightly oil a baking tray and make a layer of the artichoke hearts and asparagus. Place the salmon, skin side down, on top and pour in the white wine.

To make the crunchy topping, chop the almonds and mix with the pesto and lemon zest. Spread a layer of the mixture on top of each salmon fillet and bake for 15 minutes, or until cooked through. Season with sea salt and black pepper.

To finish, squeeze the juice from the lemon or orange over the tray, sprinkle with the dill, then serve with lemon or orange wedges and extra green veg, if you fancy it.

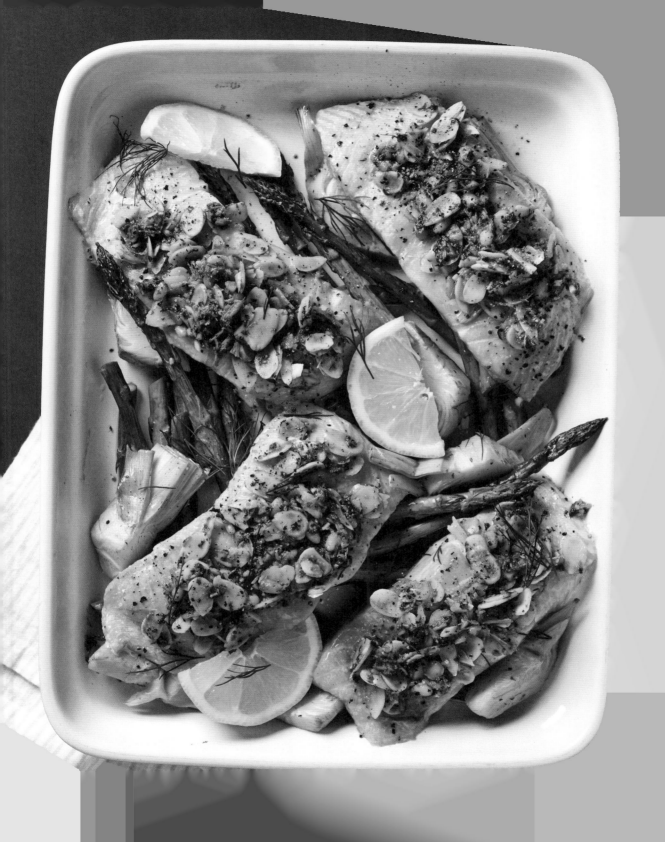

10 EXTRA ENERGY SIDES

Many of these are simple side dishes I cook for my girls, or for guests, for my husband, or even myself, during those times when my energy requirements are higher. They're all delicious, low-GI and abundantly nutritious. Most of all, they're simple.

I really believe that your Louise Parker meals should be fit for all the family – and many of you will have children, teenagers and husbands that need the extra energy that the recipes in this chapter provide. So simply add one of them on the side and you're good to go. I want to avoid your household being divided at meal times between those eating 'your food' and others eating 'family food'. I want to make your life simpler and you leaner, but also richer in time. Again, tweak away at any of these to your heart's content – the possibilities are endless.

① Honey Mustard Baby Porcupine Potatoes ⓥ

These look super-cute in baby size, but you can use larger potatoes and increase the cooking time when new potatoes are not in season. New potatoes are lower in starch than older, larger potatoes, hence I have included them here.

Serves 4 as a side

300–400g (10½–14oz) new potatoes

2 tablespoons runny honey

1 tablespoon wholegrain mustard

1 tablespoon Dijon mustard

sea salt and black pepper

3 tablespoons olive oil

Preheat the oven to 200°C/400°F/Gas Mark 6.

With a sharp knife, make a few slits sideways down each potato, keeping the nutrient-rich skin on.

Mix together the honey, mustards, seasoning and oil and, with a pastry brush, paint the glaze over the potatoes.

Place on a baking tray and bake in the middle of the oven for 25 minutes.

② Pecorino Sweet Potatoes (V)

I use pecorino here; its richer flavour means you can use less cheese, but you can substitute it with a good mature or mild Cheddar if you've got children who prefer a milder taste. This is great as a topping on any leftover minced meat, which I often spoon into little ramekins for the girls and keep in the freezer for an instant-but-healthy ready-meal.

Serves 4 as a side

2 large sweet potatoes, skin on

50–100g (½–1 cup) finely grated pecorino cheese

pinch of nutmeg

sea salt and black pepper

Preheat the oven to 200°C/425°F/Gas Mark 7.

Place the potatoes on a baking tray lined with foil in the middle of the oven (don't neglect to do this, as sweet potato juices are impossible to remove). Bake until you see the odd little black dot on the surface of the skin and the potato is very soft in the centre, about 30 minutes.

Scoop out the flesh into a bowl and add the cheese and nutmeg and mash together until you get your desired consistency. Season to taste.

③ Simple Roasted Root Veggies (Vg)

Make sure the veggie batons are the same size, so that they roast evenly. You can change up the herbs and seasoning as much as you wish. Here I've added a little orange and maple syrup, but they're perfectly gorgeous without.

Serves 4

4 large parsnips

4 large carrots

2 tablespoons olive oil

1 thyme sprig

1 teaspoon finely grated unwaxed orange zest

sea salt and black pepper

juice of 1 orange

1 tablespoon maple syrup

Preheat the oven to 220°C/425°F/Gas Mark 7.

Cut the veggies into even-sized batons, the smaller they are, the shorter the cooking time.

Mix together the olive oil, thyme, orange zest and seasoning and toss with the veggies in a roasting tin. Roast until they're golden and starting to turn a little crunchy, then remove from the oven.

Heat the orange juice in a small saucepan until it reduces a little, then add the maple syrup. Transfer the veggies to a serving platter and drizzle with the syrup.

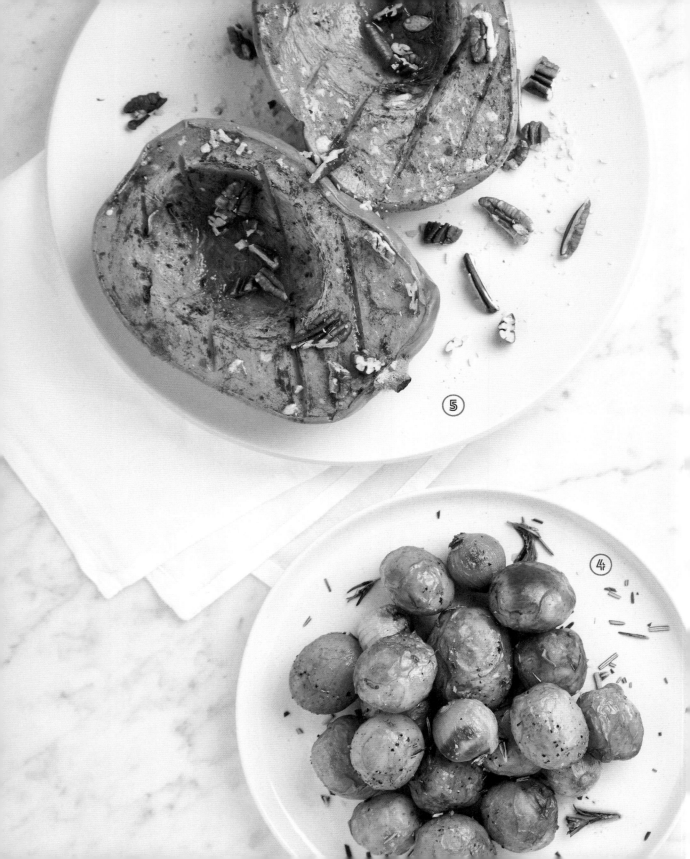

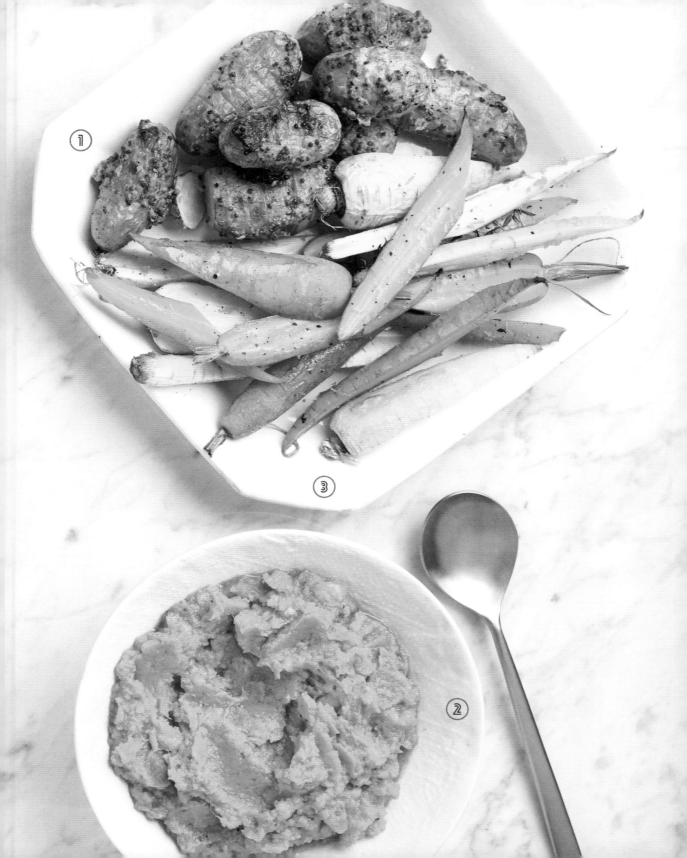

(4fr) Rosemary Roasties (Vg)

I turn to this simple dish – hardly a recipe at all – frequently, because I'm far too lazy to peel and par-boil regular roast potatoes. If I'm in a hurry, I'll double up on spuds and leave out the onions. I loathe peeling onions, so ready-peeled, frozen shallots were a happy discovery and I always keep them in the freezer. For extra indulgence, you can add some pancetta cubes; fry them off separately, blot off excess oil on kitchen paper and scatter over this wonderful side, with a good handful of chopped parsley.

Serves 4

200g (7oz) ready-peeled frozen shallots, defrosted

500g (1lb 2oz) new potatoes, skin on

2 tablespoons olive oil

1–2 rosemary sprigs, leaves stripped and chopped

sea salt and black pepper

Preheat the oven to 220°C/425°F/Gas Mark 7.

Make sure that the shallots are dry and thoroughly defrosted (pat with kitchen paper if they need some help drying). Spread the potatoes and shallots on a large baking tray, making sure that they've room to move and are not too crowded, or they won't crisp beautifully. Now simply combine the oil, rosemary and seasoning and give them a good toss.

Roast in the middle of the oven, turning occasionally, until they are evenly cooked. Depending on the size, they should take 20–30 minutes.

(5) Sweet Spiced Baked Butternut (V)

This is just heavenly. Obviously the popping candy is not essential but I love to surprise little guests with a pinch of it, that gets them giggling and begging for seconds.

Serves 4–6 as a side

2 small butternut squash

1 teaspoon ground cinnamon

½ teaspoon freshly grated nutmeg

sea salt and black pepper

2 tablespoons olive oil

100g (1 cup) pecan nuts, ready roasted and salted

1 teaspoon flavourless popping candy

Preheat the oven to 220°C/425°F/Gas Mark 7.

Cut the butternuts in half, lengthways, then remove the seeds with a spoon. Mix the cinnamon, nutmeg and seasoning into the olive oil and spread evenly over the squash halves (I use a pastry brush). Place them on a large baking tray and bake in the oven until the flesh is really soft, 30–40 minutes, depending on size.

Cut into portions if the pieces are large and keep the skin on. Sprinkle with chopped pecan nuts and, just as you are plating up, with popping candy (without telling anyone).

⑥ Funky Beets (Vg)

This instantly adds a splash of colour and flavour to anything. It works really well with pork and lamb dishes and is equally happy served hot or cold.

Serves 4

500g (1lb 2oz) beetroot

2 tablespoons olive oil

2 bulbs of garlic, cloves separated but unpeeled

3 tablespoons balsamic vinegar

sea salt and black pepper

1 teaspoon horseradish purée, to taste

chopped flat leaf parsley, to serve

feta or goats' cheese, to serve

Preheat the oven to 200°C/400°F/Gas Mark 6.

Cut each raw beetroot into eighths and arrange in an oiled roasting tin with the garlic cloves. Add 2 tablespoons of the vinegar and roast for 1 hour or until cooked.

Remove the beetroot and garlic from the roasting tin and transfer to a serving dish. Don't be tempted to discard the garlic cloves at this point, they will be beautifully sweet and gooey if you squeeze them out of their skins.

Deglaze the baking tray by adding the remaining tablespoon of balsamic vinegar and the horseradish purée and place the roasting tin over a high heat. Drizzle the sauce over the beetroot and serve, sprinkled with parsley.

Try serving this with feta or goats' cheese.

⑦ Kate's Easy Quinoa (Vg)

I use quinoa as an extra energy side. Yes, it's super-good for you, but it is comparative with brown rice in terms of nutrition. The protein is good-quality, but it's not a pure protein as we are led to believe, meaning it's great for the Lifestyle phase but not as your main source of protein. There are endless ways to jazz quinoa up, but this is perhaps my favourite. Try mixing it into My Favourite Tabbouleh (see page 114) too.

Serves 4

100g (4 packed cups) rocket, chopped

250g (9oz) ready-cooked quinoa

2 ripe avocados

juice of 1 lemon

100g (²⁄₃ cup) pomegranate seeds

2 tablespoons tahini

1 teaspoon black sesame seeds

Chop the rocket and stir into the ready-cooked quinoa. Arrange on a plate, with slices of avocado (drenched in lemon juice to stop them going brown).

Sprinkle with pomegranate seeds and drizzle with tahini and some black sesame seeds to serve.

The Girls' Favourite Coconut Rice (Vg)

I started cooking this as a way to nudge my girls into choosing brown rice over basmati, by adding delicious coconut milk and pineapple. Now they are happy to eat brown rice plain, but this is a lovely special side to do from time to time. I always freeze it in portions, so I have it on hand. I know you're not meant to freeze rice, but my mother has always done it and now, so do I. I insist you use US cups here (1 cup = 250ml), as cooking perfect rice is purely about ratios.

Season with fresh herbs, if you like; I love Thai basil or mint here.

Serves 4

1 tablespoon coconut oil, plus more for the pineapple

1½ cups brown rice

2 cups coconut milk

2 cups water

1 tablespoon unsweetened desiccated coconut

pinch of sea salt

400g (14oz) pineapple, cut into fingers

2 tablespoons shredded coconut, toasted

Melt the coconut oil in a saucepan and spread it out evenly over the base of the pan, then remove from the heat. Rinse the rice and add to the pan, along with the coconut milk, water, desiccated coconut and salt. Now bring to the boil, then immediately reduce the heat to a simmer and clap the lid on. Cook until all the liquid is absorbed (40–50 minutes depending on the rice you use).

Meanwhile, coat the pineapple with coconut oil and cook on a very hot griddle pan until striped on both sides.

Fluff up the rice with a fork and serve topped with the griddled pineapple and sprinkled with the toasted coconut.

⑨ Wild Rice with Pomegranate Ⓥg

Wild rice can take up to 40–50 minutes to cook. I boil it as I would pasta, in plenty of boiling water.

Serves 4–6

360g (2 cups) wild rice

1 litre (4 cups) water

½ vegetable bouillon cube

100g (3½ cups) kale, coarse stalks discarded, chopped (or use spinach)

1 tablespoon walnut oil

juice of 1 lemon

100g (⅔ cup) pomegranate seeds

2 tablespoons walnuts, toasted

sea salt and black pepper

Rinse the wild rice and place in a saucepan with the water and bouillon cube. Bring it to the boil, then reduce the heat to a simmer, lid off. Keep an eye on it and as soon as it is cooked, strain in a sieve. Make sure it is fully drained and dry before assembling the dish.

While the rice is still warm, add the kale and allow it to wilt a little. Add the walnut oil and lemon juice, stir, then top with the pomegranate seeds and walnuts. Season well to taste.

⑩ Milly's Winter Mash Ⓥ

This is the best mash. I've included sweet potato, which has a lower GI than large whites and the carrots and parsnips just add more nutrition and depth of flavour. If you don't like raw onion you can caramelize it in a little olive oil over a low heat.

Serves 4–6

2 carrots

2 parsnips

2 large white potatoes

2 sweet potatoes

½ vegetable bouillon cube

1 red onion, finely sliced

1 teaspoon red wine vinegar

sea salt and black pepper

1 tablespoon butter

1 tablespoon single or double cream

50g (½ cup) finely grated Parmesan cheese, plus more shavings to serve

50g (½ cup) grated mature Cheddar cheese

Peel and very roughly chop the vegetables to the same size. Boil in plenty of water and the vegetable bouillon over a medium heat until they are just cooked.

Meanwhile, combine the onion and vinegar and season to taste.

Drain the vegetables well and mash, along with the butter, cream and both cheeses. Top the mash with the onions and a few Parmesan shavings.

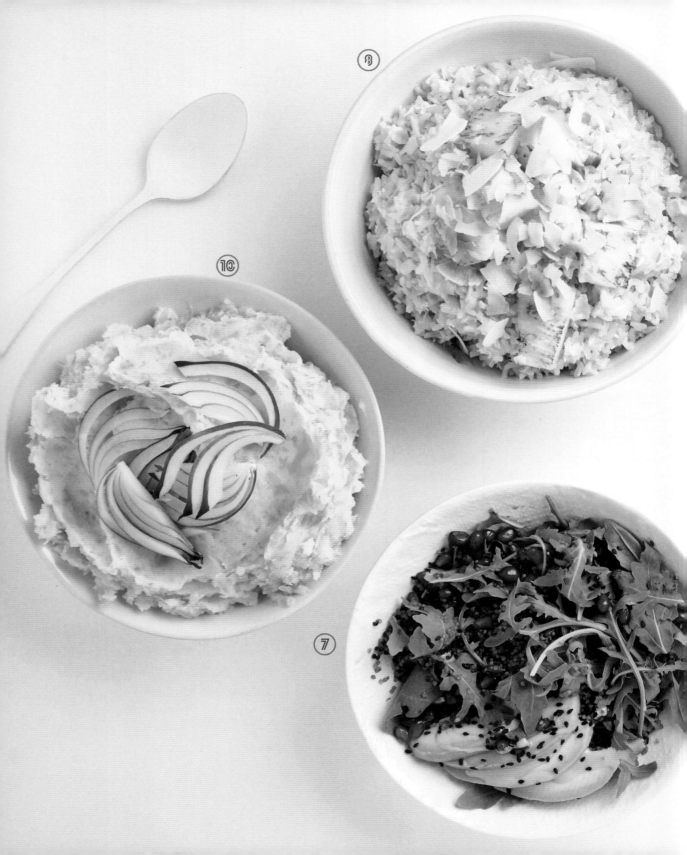

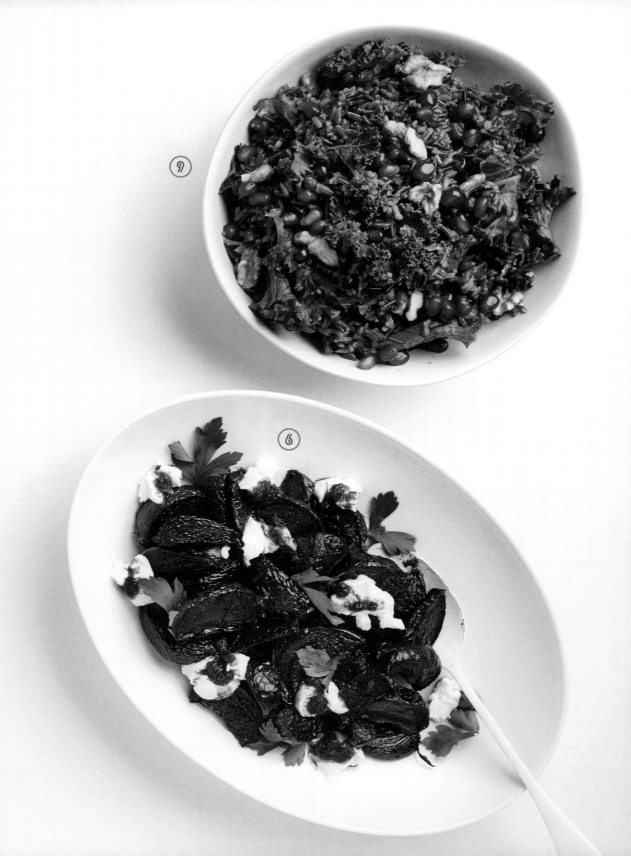

7

FOOD FOR FRIENDS

Luckily, my friends are pretty low-maintenance and I tend not to throw fancy dinner parties. But if I do have a gathering or a celebration where I want to pull something a little more loving and gorgeous out of the oven, here are just some of my favourites. And you don't have to spend a fortune. Yes, there are a small scattering of luxe ingredients here, but most are just regular, inexpensive foods cooked cleverly, or with extra care, or with a few fancy embellishments. Don't forget that once you're in the Lifestyle Phase and eating to the Method just 70–80 per cent of the time, you can serve whatever you want at a dinner party. But while you're in the Transform phase, these are the dishes for you when you're entertaining: your guests won't even realize the food is good for them.

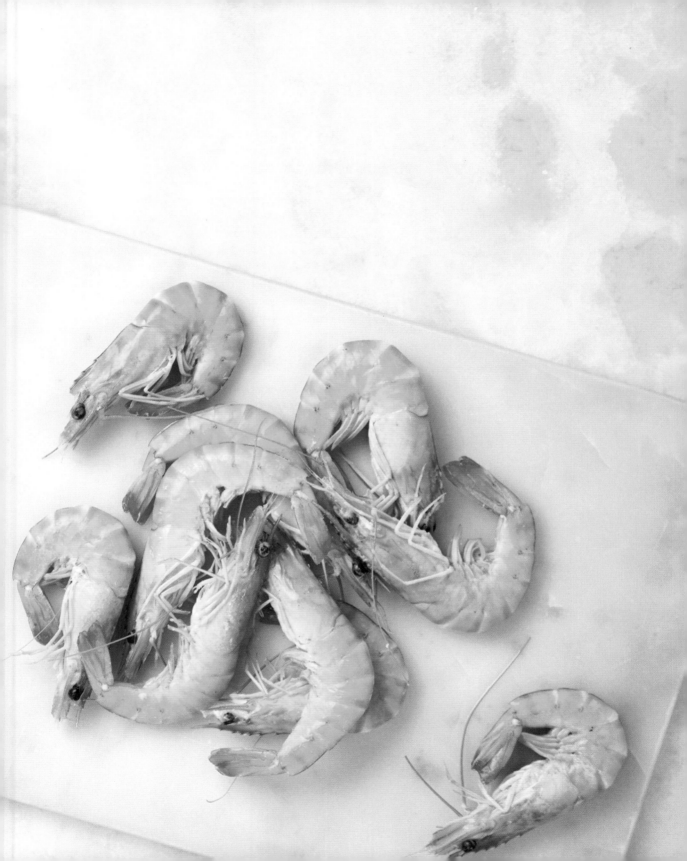

Cajun Steak with Herb & Lime Slaw

Serves 4

FOR THE STEAKS

4 x 150g (5½oz) fillet steaks

1 tablespoon Cajun seasoning

1 teaspoon sea salt

1 teaspoon black pepper

1 tablespoon mild olive oil

FOR THE SLAW

¼ head of red cabbage,
very finely sliced

¼ head of Savoy cabbage,
very finely sliced

2 carrots, shredded with a mandolin,
or spiralized

8 radishes, finely sliced

good handful of flat leaf parsley
leaves, chopped

good handful of coriander leaves,
chopped

2 tablespoons mild olive oil

juice of 2 limes (roll on a hard surface
before you squeeze)

2 tablespoons toasted pine nuts

You can use any steak here: sirloin, fillet, ribeye, or my most recent obsession, bavette, which is a classic French cut absolutely full of flavour and really good value. Most good supermarkets stock some wonderful ready-made rubs; do experiment with different flavours. You can prepare the slaw and season the steaks earlier in the day, adding the lime juice just before serving. I sometimes slice the steaks thickly and serve on a bed of slaw, or more casually on the table on a big board, with everyone helping themselves. In the summer it makes a great outdoor barbecue meal.

Remove the steaks from the fridge and allow them to come to room temperature.

Mix the Cajun seasoning, salt and pepper into the olive oil and massage over the steaks really well. Allow them to rest if you have time, ideally for 10 minutes.

Meanwhile, make the slaw. Simply combine all the vegetables and herbs in a bowl and mix well.

When you're ready to eat, heat a large griddle pan, without oil, over a very high heat. Now simply fry the steaks. The time will depend on the cut: the thicker the cut, the longer you will need to cook the meat on each side. It'll vary between 2–5 minutes, depending on how well cooked you like them. Allow them to rest, covered in foil, for at least 5 minutes before serving.

Meanwhile dress the slaw with the olive oil, salt and pepper and plenty of lime juice. Sprinkle with warm, toasted pine nuts just before serving with the rested steaks.

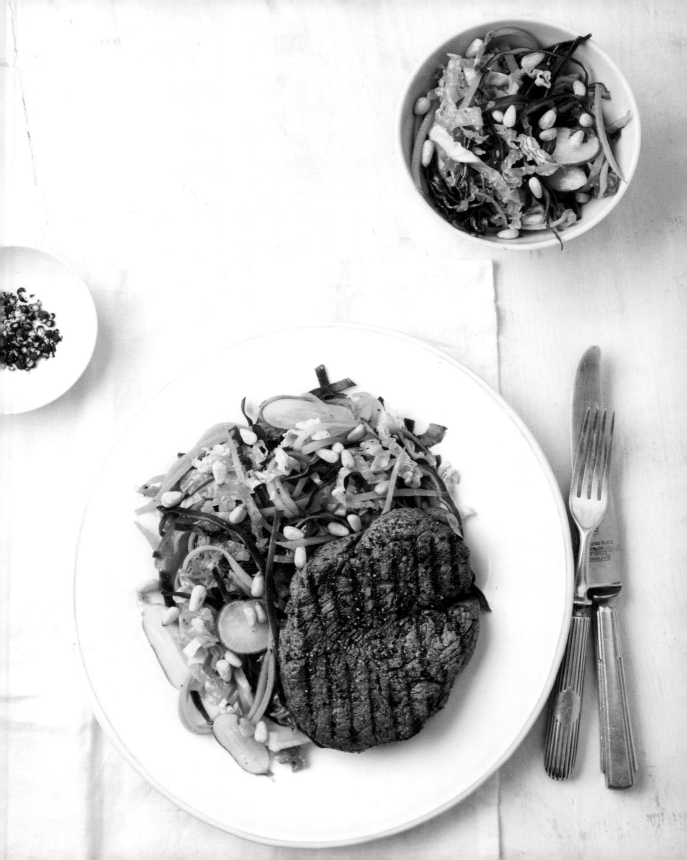

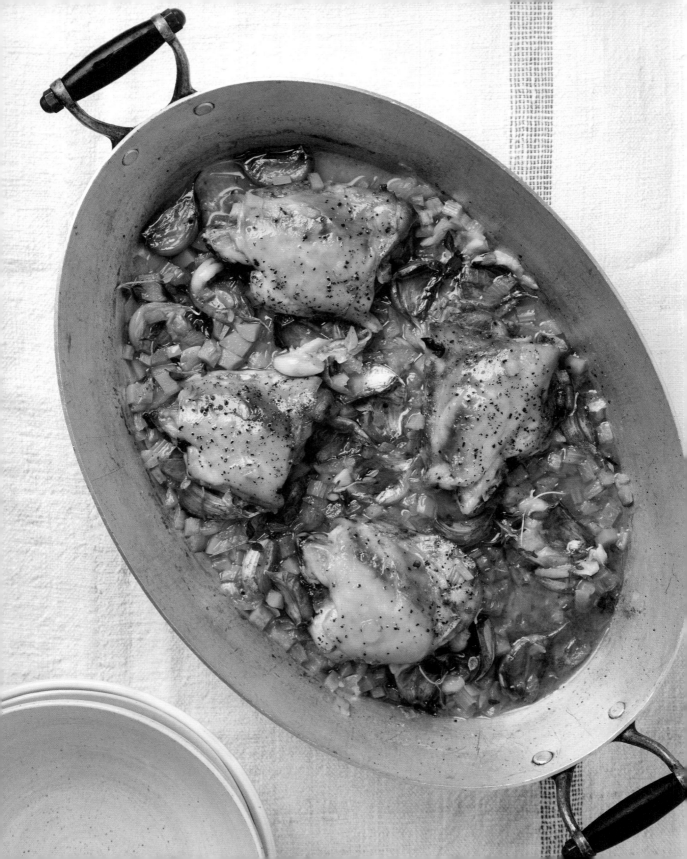

Chicken with Four Bulbs of Garlic

Serves 4

2 tablespoons olive oil

8 skinless, bone-in chicken thighs

1 large onion, finely chopped

1 celery stick, finely chopped

1 carrot, finely chopped

40–50 garlic cloves, skin on, from 4 whole garlic bulbs

100ml (scant ½ cup) dry white wine

100ml (scant ½ cup) Cognac, or brandy

3 thyme sprigs

sea salt and black pepper

There are many versions of this French classic, and I've leaned it out as much as I can while ensuring it retains its rich, sweet, comforting deliciousness. Don't be put off by the amount of garlic. I love it with simply steamed spinach, but it's also gorgeous with my cauliflower cream (see page 128).

Preheat the oven to 160°C/325°F/Gas Mark 3.

Heat 1 tablespoon of the oil in a casserole dish over a medium heat and slowly brown the chicken thighs on all sides. As the skin is removed, you'll need to do this over a lower temperature than usual and give them a good wiggle around to prevent them sticking to the dish.

Remove the chicken from the dish and sweat the onion, celery and carrot in the remaining tablespoon of olive oil until the onion is nicely softened. Return the chicken to the dish with all the garlic cloves – do not panic – and add the wine, Cognac and thyme sprigs. Season. Give it a gentle stir, scraping up any bits from the bottom of the dish without upsetting the chicken too much, then pop in the oven for 1 hour and 30 minutes, until the chicken just falls off the bone and the garlic is sticky and sweet. Check the seasoning and adjust if necessary.

Serve in large bowls, on a bed of steamed or sautéed spinach.

Roast Prawns with Puy lentils

Use ready-cooked Puy lentils if you're in a hurry; just make sure that you add plenty of seasoning and a dash of champagne or white wine vinegar to replace the wine.

Serves 4

FOR THE LENTILS

1 teaspoon olive oil

1 onion, finely chopped

1 carrot, finely chopped

1 celery stick, finely chopped

300g (1½ cups) Puy lentils

600ml (2½ cups) vegetable stock

600ml (2½ cups) water

200ml (¾ cup) white wine

sea salt and black pepper

2 heads of Cos lettuce, finely sliced

FOR THE PRAWNS

400g (14oz) prawns, shell on

1 tablespoon olive oil

2 garlic cloves, finely chopped

chopped coriander leaves, to serve

2 red chillies, finely chopped, to serve

FOR THE DRESSING

1 garlic clove, crushed

1 tablespoon each of soy sauce, rice wine vinegar, olive oil and sesame oil

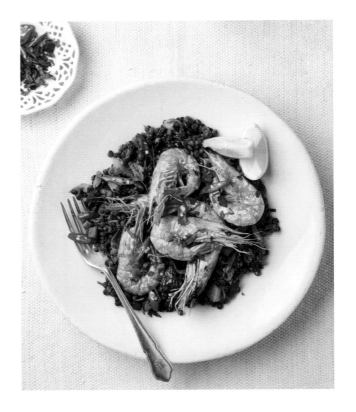

Heat the olive oil in a pan over a medium heat and gently fry the onion, carrot and celery until soft. Wash and drain the lentils and add to the pan with the stock, water and wine. Bring to the boil, then reduce the heat and simmer for 20 minutes. Once cooked, season to taste and stir in the sliced lettuce until wilted.

Meanwhile, for the prawns, preheat the oven to 220°C/425°F/Gas Mark 7 and line a baking tray with foil. Lay on the prawns, brush with the olive oil and sprinkle with the garlic and salt and pepper, then bake in the oven for 8 minutes.

Mix the dressing ingredients together. Serve the prawns on top of the lentils, drizzle with the dressing and garnish with chopped coriander and red chillies.

Ceviche

Make sure you use really fresh ingredients for this Peruvian dish as the fish and seafood aren't cooked over heat, they are marinated in the citrus juices. It's a great way to really preserve the flavour of top quality seafood and makes a zingy and fresh meal that looks like you've made lots of effort.

Serves 4

FOR THE CEVICHE

600g (1lb 5oz) very fresh cod, monkfish and/or scallops

juice of 4 limes

1 garlic clove, finely chopped

sea salt and black pepper

2 green chillies, finely chopped

1 shallot, finely chopped

4 tablespoons chopped coriander leaves

2 baby red peppers, finely chopped

2 baby yellow peppers, finely chopped

FOR THE CHOPPED SALAD

2 heads of Romaine lettuce, finely chopped

2 ripe avocados, finely chopped

2 tablespoons chopped flat leaf parsley leaves

2 tablespoons chopped coriander leaves

2 spring onions, sliced lengthways

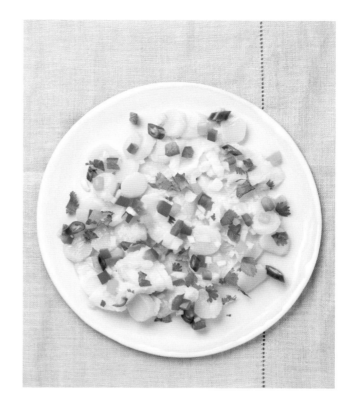

Cut the seafood into fine slices or little chunks and place in a flat dish, covering with the lime juice, garlic, salt and pepper. Cover and marinate in the fridge for 3 hours. Remove and add the remaining ingredients, cover once more and return to the fridge for a further 3 hours.

When you're ready to eat, mix together all the ingredients for the chopped salad and serve alongside the ceviche.

Herbed Rack of Lamb with Heirloom Tomato & Feta Salad

Serves 4

FOR THE LAMB AND HERB CRUST

crust of 1 slice of wholemeal bread

leaves from a small bunch of
flat leaf parsley

leaves from a small bunch of mint

leaves from 1 rosemary sprig

leaves from 1 thyme sprig

1 teaspoon sea salt

½ teaspoon black pepper

1 tablespoon olive oil

50g (½ cup) finely grated
Parmesan cheese

1 × 8-rib rack of lamb

FOR THE SALAD

200g (7oz) green or yellow heirloom
tomatoes, chopped

200g (7oz) red or orange heirloom
tomatoes, chopped

good bunch of mint leaves, finely
chopped, plus extra to garnish

good bunch of flat leaf parsley leaves,
finely chopped

½ cucumber, deseeded and sliced

juice of 1 lemon

100g (1 cup) crumbled feta cheese

There are endless rubs and toppings that you can use for a rack of lamb, but this super-simple seasoning is the one I turn to most. Try to buy the lamb already 'French-trimmed' and prepared for you. Each portion is two ribs, or three for a hungry man. You may want to remove the visible fat when eating, but keep it on when you roast it for a fuller flavour. This works beautifully with a fresh salad in the summer, or any of my warm vegetables in the winter months.

Preheat the oven to 240°C/475°F/Gas Mark 9.

To prepare the herb crust, throw all the ingredients into a blender and whizz for 1 minute, until you've a bright green, textured crumb topping.

Cover the rack of lamb generously with the herb crust, and place in the middle of the oven, reducing the oven temperature as you do so to 190°C/375°F/Gas Mark 5. Depending on how rare you like it, a rack of 8 ribs will take 20–30 minutes. If you like it pink inside, as I do, aim for 20 minutes.

Meanwhile, prepare the salad by simply combining the tomatoes, herbs and cucumber, dressing it generously with lemon juice and crumbled feta cheese.

Remove the lamb from the oven and allow it to rest for 10 minutes, covered in foil, to keep the meat really juicy.

Carve the racks of lamb between the ribs and serve alongside the salad.

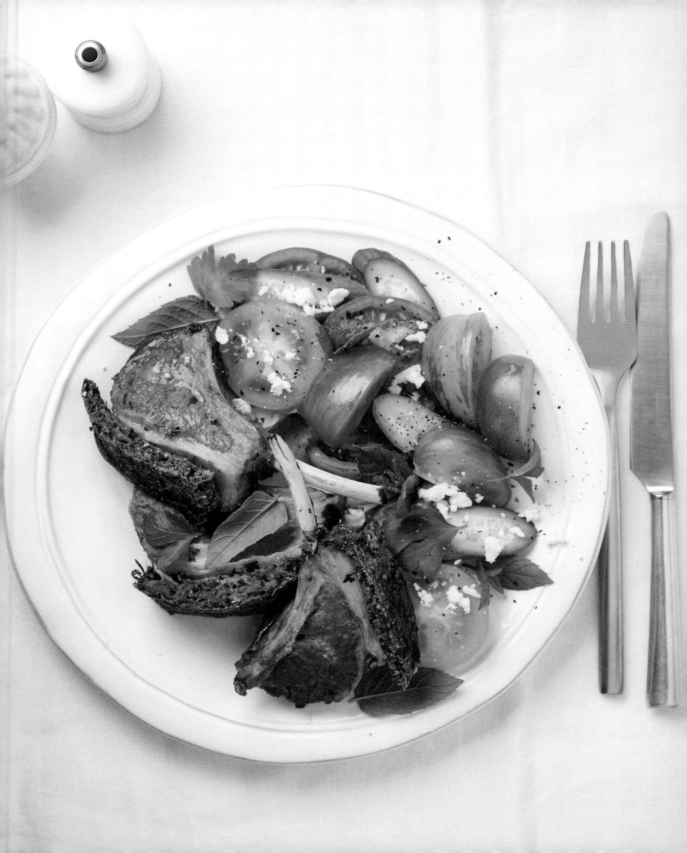

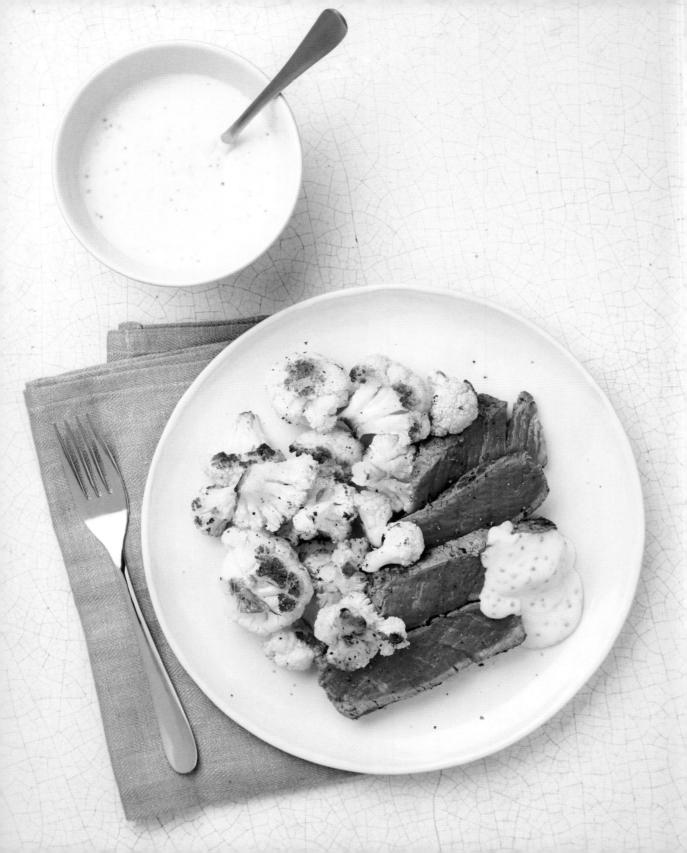

Roast Fillet of Beef with Roast Cauliflower & Mustard Sauce

Serves 6

FOR THE CAULIFLOWER

1½ cauliflowers, cut into florets

1½ tablespoons olive oil

sea salt and black pepper

FOR THE BEEF

800g (1lb 12oz) fillet of beef

1 tablespoon olive oil

FOR THE SAUCE

2 tablespoons mustard seeds

½ tablespoon olive oil

1 teaspoon English mustard

1 tablespoons Dijon mustard

4 tablespoons full-fat crème fraîche

4 tablespoons 0% Greek yogurt

juice of 2 lemons, plus a pinch of finely grated unwaxed lemon zest

This is a posh crowd-pleaser when you need a luxe-but-foolproof meal. Serve with a fresh green salad in the summer – finishing the roast off on a barbecue – or serve with hot green veggies in the winter. While this will serve six, I often double up so that I've got tender, cold beef for leftovers, which are perfect for my Ten-minute Thai Beef Salad (see page 162).

Preheat the oven to 240°C/475°F/Gas Mark 9.

First, tumble the cauliflower florets into a roasting tin and cover well with the oil, 1 teaspoon of salt and ½ teaspoon of black pepper. Place in the bottom of the oven and roast for 35 minutes until golden.

Pat the beef dry with kitchen paper and rub well with the olive oil, 2 teaspoons more salt and 1 teaspoon more black pepper.

Now for the sauce. Fry the mustard seeds in the oil in a saucepan over a medium heat – lid on or they will pop all over the kitchen – for 2 minutes. Remove the seeds and set aside. Increase the heat to high and sear the beef on all sides until browned.

Place the joint in a roasting dish in the middle of the oven and cook for 20 minutes for medium rare.

While the cauliflower and beef are in the oven, finish the sauce. Combine all the ingredients except the mustard seeds in a bowl and whisk, adding the mustard seeds once they have cooled. Taste and adjust the seasoning.

Once cooked, allow the beef to rest, covered with foil, for 15 minutes.

Carve and serve alongside the roasted cauliflower, drizzled with the mustard cream.

Slow-roast Moroccan Lamb with Butter Bean Purée

Serves 8, with leftovers (your portion of lamb should be roughly 175g/6oz of meat)

FOR THE LAMB

8 red onions, halved

2 garlic bulbs, halved widthways

2kg (4lb 8oz) leg of lamb, on the bone

2 tablespoons ras el hanout

2 teaspoons sea salt

1 tablespoon olive oil

16 baby aubergines, halved

200g (1 cup) cherry tomatoes

200g (7oz) green beans, trimmed and halved

200ml (scant 1 cup) water

dried rose petals (optional, of course!)

a few mint leaves, sliced

FOR THE BUTTER BEAN PURÉE

4 x 400g (14oz) cans butter beans, drained and rinsed

2 tablespoons tahini

2 tablespoons olive oil

1 teaspoon sea salt

½ teaspoon black pepper

1 roasted garlic bulb (see above)

This is a recipe I've cooked perhaps 100 times as it really is foolproof and perfect for Sunday lunch with a crowd of hungry friends. Mr P has many skills, but carving is not one of them, so the fact that the meat just falls off the bone is a bonus. The meat cooks for so long that the fat will just drain off, yet the meat is so utterly tender and delicious.

Preheat the oven to 160°C/325°F/Gas Mark 3.

Throw the onions and garlic into a roasting tin and place the lamb on top. Cover well with foil, sealing around the tin and making sure there are no gaps. Roast for 2 hours. You can baste it every half hour or so, but you could equally go out for a walk and leave it and it will look after itself.

Remove 1 garlic bulb from the tin for the butter bean purée. Mix the ras el hanout and salt into the olive oil to form a paste and brush over the lamb, ensuring you cover the sides too. Pop back into the oven, foil off this time, and cook for a further hour. Finally add the baby aubergines, tomatoes, green beans and water to the roasting tin and return to the oven for another hour.

Remove from the oven, cover in foil, and leave to rest for 30 minutes. Meanwhile, prepare the butter bean purée. Place the beans, tahini, olive oil, salt and pepper in a food processor, squeeze the roasted garlic cloves out of their skins to join them, then blend until really smooth and creamy. Test for seasoning and add a little water if you'd like a lighter consistency.

Serve the lamb shredded over the butter bean purée on a large platter. Remove the garlic cloves and the red onions if you wish, and spoon the gooey veggies over the meat. Sprinkle with rose petals (if you like) and mint to serve.

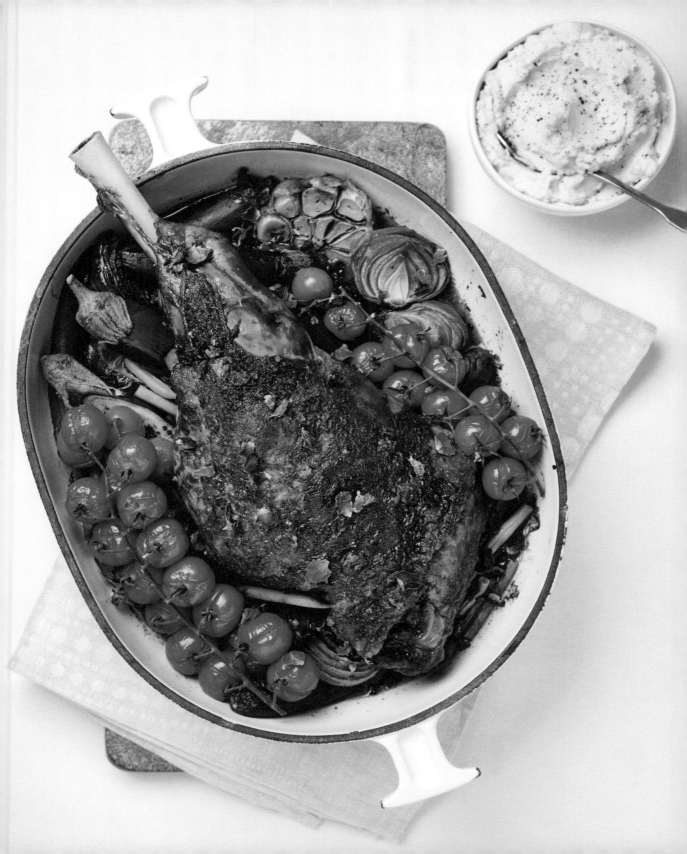

Monkfish Tandoor

This wonderful marinade is the perfect quick-fix cheat – hardly a recipe at all.

Serves 4

FOR THE VEGGIES

2 teaspoons light olive oil

2 teaspoons cumin seeds

1 garlic clove, crushed or very finely chopped

450g (1lb) young leaf spinach

200g (7oz) chard

sea salt and black pepper

FOR THE MARINADE

4 garlic cloves, grated

2 teaspoons grated fresh root ginger

4 tablespoons full-fat Greek yogurt

1 tablespoon tandoori paste

1 teaspoon chickpea flour

handful of coriander leaves, chopped

1–2 red chillies, to taste

FOR THE FISH

800g (1lb 12oz) monkfish, cut into chunks

juice of ½ lemon or lime

pinch of sea salt

1 tablespoon ghee

TO GARNISH

Raita (see page 138)

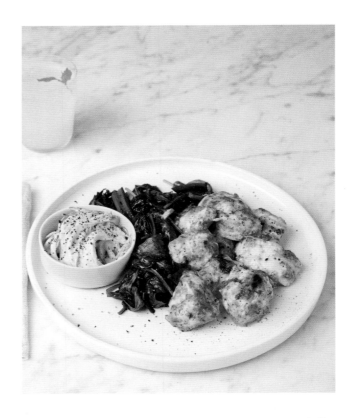

Mix together the marinade ingredients in a non-metallic dish. Place the monkfish into the dish and coat well with the marinade. Leave to marinate for at least 2 hours.

Preheat the oven to 220°C/425°F/Gas Mark 7.

Remove the monkfish from the marinade and place in an ovenproof dish. Bake until cooked through, about 10 minutes.

In a wok, heat the oil over a medium heat and fry the cumin seeds for 30 seconds, then add the garlic for 15 seconds and now, bit by bit, add the spinach and chard, and stir until wilted. Season well.

Serve the baked monkfish with the wilted greens and raita on the side.

Konstantin's Miso Cod

Thank you to Rob and Konstantin for sharing this with us. Rob is a walking advert for our Method and luckily his boyfriend is the most wonderful chef.

Serves 4

FOR THE DRESSING

100g (⅔ cup) sesame seeds

2 tablespoons toasted sesame oil

1 tablespoon Japanese rice vinegar

pinch of stevia

2 tablespoons natural yogurt

FOR THE COD

4 cod loin fillets, each about 150g (5½oz)

3 tablespoons good miso paste

2 teaspoons sesame oil

800g (1lb 12oz) spinach, coarse stalks discarded

200g (1½ cups) frozen shelled edamame beans

2 spring onions, sliced

1 red chilli, sliced

1 teaspoon chopped coriander leaves

1 teaspoon black sesame seeds

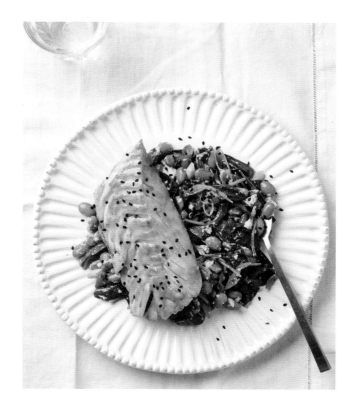

Preheat the oven to 200°C/400°F/Gas Mark 6 while you prepare the dressing.

Using a pestle and mortar, crush the sesame seeds and stir in the sesame oil, rice vinegar and stevia until you've got a thick paste. Now stir in the yogurt and set aside.

Coat the cod fillets in the miso paste, wrap in foil and bake for 20 minutes.

Now heat the sesame oil in a pan over a medium heat and sauté the spinach and edamame beans until the spinach wilts and the edamame are defrosted. Add the dressing, spring onions, chilli and chopped coriander and stir through.

Serve the miso cod on top of the vegetables and sprinkled with sesame seeds.

Lobster with Lime Butter & Zesty Spring Vegetables

Serves 4

FOR THE SALAD

150g (5½oz) tenderstem broccoli

150g (5½oz) fine French beans

150g (5½oz) baby carrots

FOR THE LOBSTER

finely grated zest and juice of
1 unwaxed lime

handful of chopped flat leaf
parsley leaves

sea salt and black pepper

100g (scant ½ cup) unsalted butter,
softened

8 small or 4 large lobsters, shell on,
halved and cleaned

good handful of chopped dill

sprinkle of chilli flakes

FOR THE DRESSING

2 tablespoons olive oil

2 garlic cloves, smashed

1 strip of unwaxed lime zest,
plus juice of 1 lime

1 teaspoon Dijon mustard

Before you roll your eyes at the expense, low-cost supermarkets now sell lobster for the price of chicken, so stock up. I can't get enough of this and always keep the shells to make a rich fish stock to freeze for a later date.

Blanch all the vegetables for the salad in boiling water for 4–5 minutes, then transfer immediately to a large bowl of cold water and ice cubes for 2 minutes to stop the cooking. Drain.

Preheat the grill to high. Mix the lime zest, parsley and salt and pepper into the butter and spread evenly over the cut sides of the lobsters. Place under a hot grill and grill, flesh side down, for 3 minutes. Turn, coat again with the butter mix and grill for a further 3–5 minutes until cooked through and nicely browned.

For the dressing, heat the olive oil, garlic and lime zest over a very low heat for 1 minute. Remove the zest and garlic, season to taste and whisk in the lime juice and mustard. Toss through the blanched veggies.

Place the lobsters on a large platter surrounded by the dressed veggies. Sprinkle with dill and chilli flakes and serve.

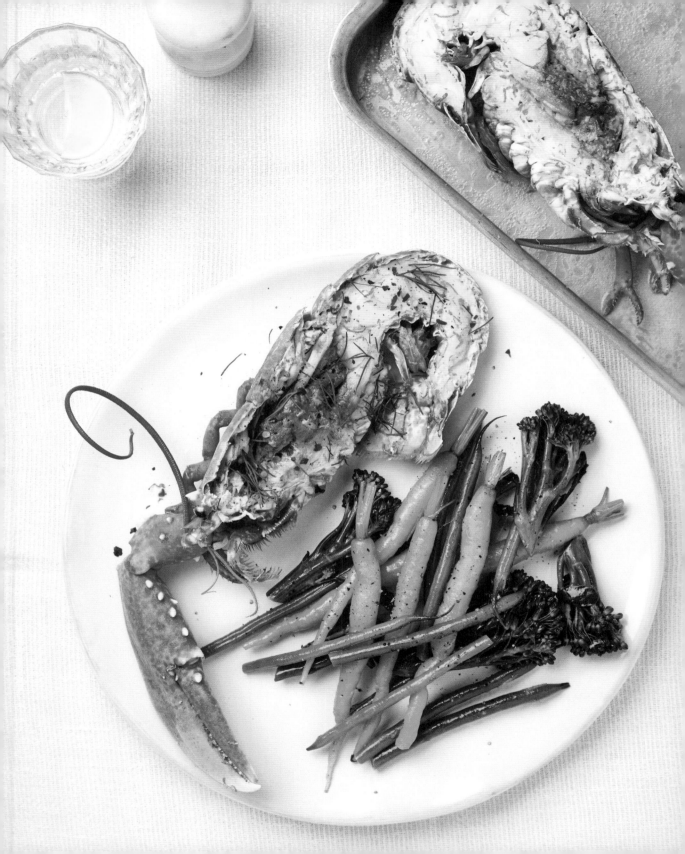

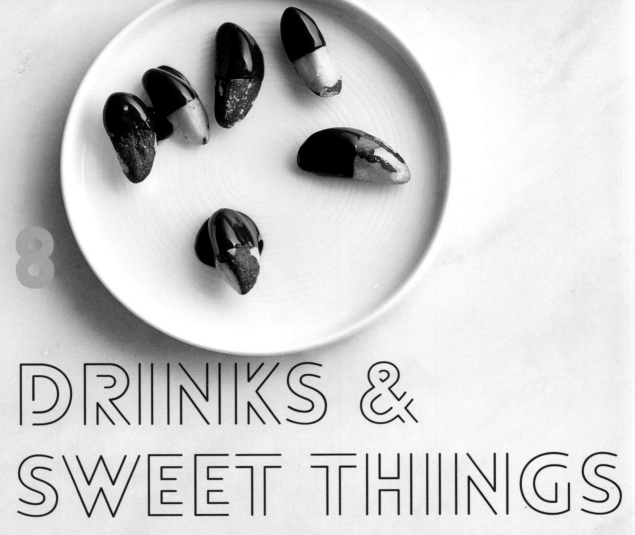

8

DRINKS & SWEET THINGS

As you know, my approach is sugar-free. But only until you reach your goal and then, when you're in the Lifestyle Phase, you can have that chocolate bombe and enjoy it guilt-free… just in balance. What I really hate are hidden sugars (such as the dates and honey in 'natural, gluten-free' bars) that basically kid you into thinking you're eating something that will reduce the size of your backside. Sugar is sugar, whether it's natural or not.

However, here is a little section for you, for those days when you just need to curl up and have something sweet. Some have reduced sugar and others are sugar-free.

And remember, once you're at goal, you will be able to eat crème brûlée again – it's just that I'd rather you did that mindfully, than unknowingly eat the same amount of sugar in an 'organically overweight' bar (see page 14).

Enjoy a little sweetness, although you'll probably find that you desire less the more you live our Method. There are some great options here too for your family – my girls love the sugar-free hot chocolate! My favourite is the thick Mexican Hot Chocolate (see page 207), drunk while cuddled up on the sofa with a blanket, fire on.

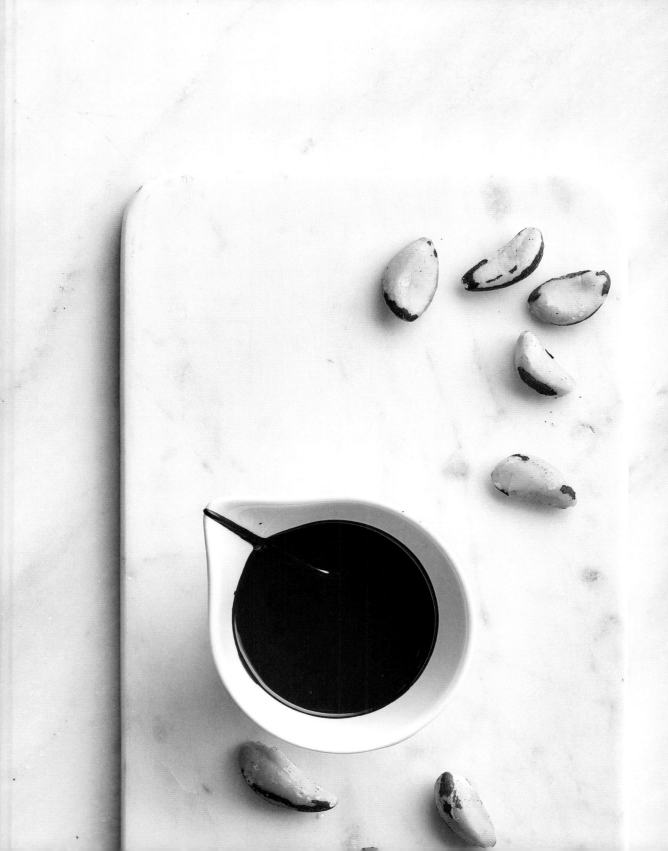

Grilled Apricots & Passion Fruit ⓥ

Most stone fruits are just divine when grilled – they caramelize and the grilling brings slightly unripe fruit to life. Chop and change and leave out the stevia if you don't need the sweetness.

Serves 2

4 apricots, halved

1 teaspoon unsalted butter, melted

pulp of 2 passion fruits

pinch of stevia, to taste

1 tablespoon toasted flaked almonds

Brush the cut sides of the apricots with a little butter and place, flat sides down, on to a hot, non-stick griddle pan. Leave them alone for 2–3 minutes.

Meanwhile, taste the passion fruit pulp and add stevia if you'd like it sweeter.

Serve the apricots drizzled with the passion fruit pulp, sprinkled with warm toasted flaked almonds.

Grilled Pineapple & Vanilla Ricotta ⓥ

I often use ready-bought fresh rings to save time, then you can throw this together in minutes. The fragrance is just insanely good. Let it grill until it's almost charred so that the fruit is firm but sticky.

Serves 4

600g (1lb 5oz) peeled pineapple, sliced into 8 rings

1 teaspoon unsalted butter, melted

120g (½ cup) ricotta cheese

½ teaspoon vanilla paste

4 walnuts, preferably roasted and salted

Brush the pineapple rings with a little butter and place on a hot, non-stick griddle pan for 1 minute each side, until you've got lovely stripy lines.

Meanwhile, mix the ricotta with the vanilla.

Serve 2 pineapple rings per person, with the ricotta cream alongside, sprinkled with chopped or whole roasted and salted walnuts.

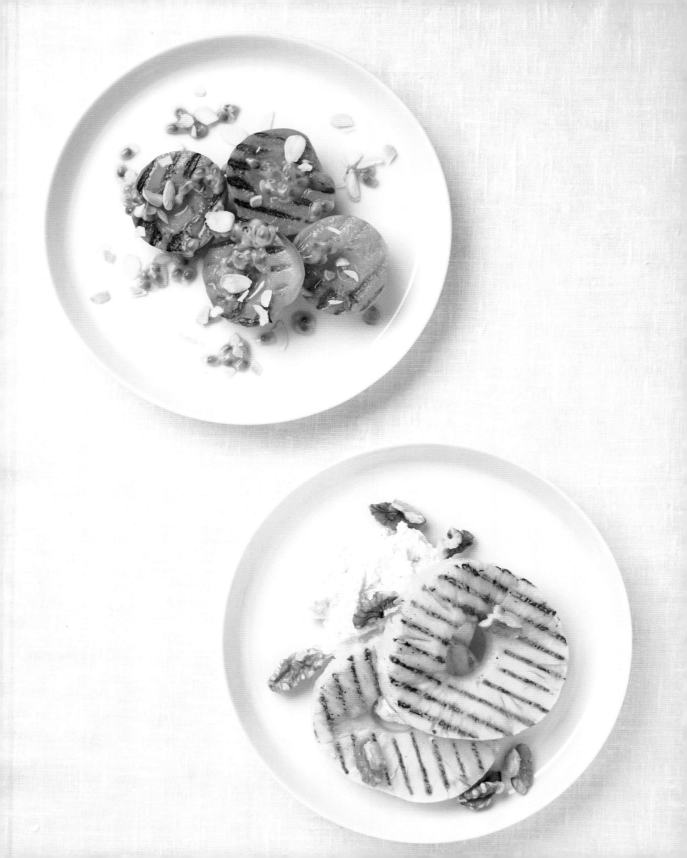

FROZEN YOGURTS

There are endless varieties of sugar-free frozen yogurts that you can make. The results will be slightly firmer using a mini ice-cream maker (in which case, blend until smooth and runny and then add to the machine), or just use a powerful blender such as a Vitamix. The trick is to blend very quickly – just until the ingredients come together – or it will over-melt. If it does, pop it into the freezer for 10 minutes to firm up again.

① Summer Berry ⓥ

Serves 4

250g (1½ cups) frozen summer berries

250g (1 cup) 0% Greek yogurt

½ teaspoon stevia, or to taste

4 teaspoons dried strawberries

4 mint sprigs

Place all the ingredients except the dried strawberries and mint in a powerful blender. Set it to high speed and, using the tamper, push the berries down towards the blade. It should take 20–30 seconds to come together.

Spoon into bowls and decorate each bowl with 1 teaspoon of dried strawberries and a mint sprig.

② Mango & Pistachio ⓥ

Serves 4

250g (1½ cups) frozen mango

250g (1 cup) 0% Greek yogurt

4 teaspoons chopped salted pistachios

Place the mango and yogurt in a powerful blender. Set it to high speed and, using the tamper, push the mango cubes down towards the blade. It should take 20–30 seconds to come together to a creamy consistency.

Spoon into bowls and decorate with the chopped pistachios.

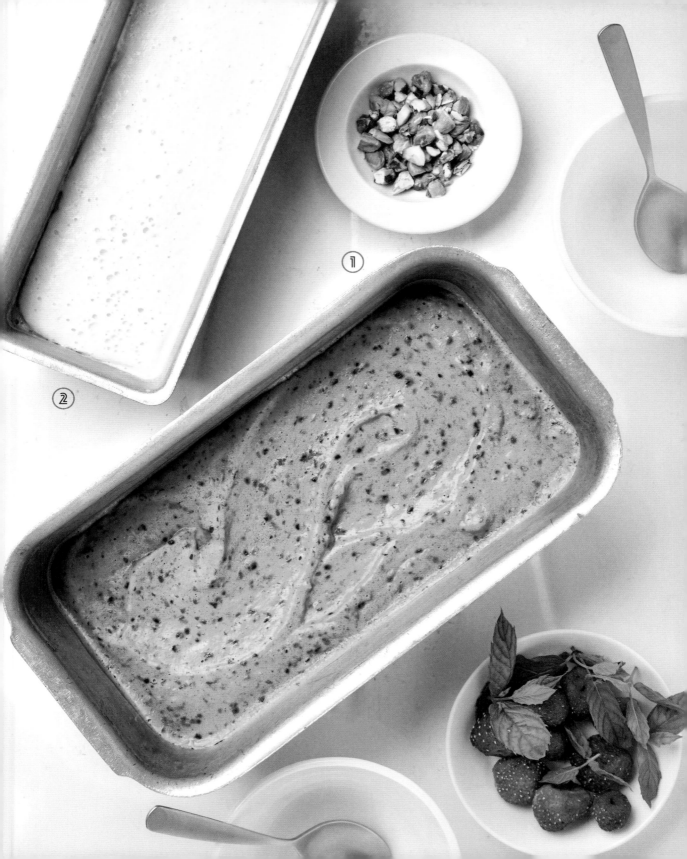

CHOCOLATE 3 WAYS

You asked, I listened. During Transform, use common sense and don't go overboard. Remember that when you're in your best body, you'll be eating whatever you want 30 per cent of the time anyway – so chocolate bombes await. In the meantime, here's a few ideas that will get you over that chocolate craving that invariably hits us all from time to time.

① Chocolate-dipped Brazils Ⓥ

For variety, leave out the raspberries and sea salt and try chilli flakes too, or chopped roasted nuts.

Makes 20 (2–4 per person)

150g (5½oz) dark chocolate, 70% cocoa solids

20 whole Brazil nuts

2 tablespoons dried raspberries

sea salt (optional)

Place a heatproof bowl over a saucepan of simmering water; the bowl should not touch the surface of the water.

Break or chop the chocolate roughly, place it in the bowl and melt, keeping the heat very low.

Once it has melted, dip half the nuts into the chocolate, then sprinkle with the raspberry pieces and just a couple of flakes of sea salt, if desired.

Place on greaseproof paper and pop in the fridge to set. They will keep in an airtight container for up to a week, although the chances of them lasting that long are slim…

② Hot Chocolate Ⓥ

You can add a pinch of good coffee granules to intensify the cocoa flavour here, if you want.

Serves 1

200ml (¾ cup) semi-skimmed (1 or 2%) milk, or soya milk

1 heaped teaspoon cocoa powder

½ teaspoon vanilla paste

stevia, to taste

Heat the milk in a saucepan over a medium-low heat, just until steaming.

Mix the cocoa powder into 1 tablespoon of boiling water in a mug, to make a smooth paste. Add the vanilla and stevia to taste

Top up with hot milk and stir. I like to do this using my milk frother for a creamier hot chocolate.

③ Mexican Hot Chocolate ⓥ

I adore this recipe. But you can experiment with different quantities of spices, or try using chilli flakes instead of cayenne pepper.

Serves 1

1 heaped teaspoon cocoa powder

¼ teaspoon cornflour

pinch of ground cinnamon

pinch of ground nutmeg

pinch of cayenne pepper

½ teaspoon vanilla paste

stevia, to taste

200ml (¾ cup) semi-skimmed (1 or 2%) milk, or soya milk

Mix all the ingredients except the milk with 1 tablespoon of boiling water to make a very smooth paste.

Pour the milk into a saucepan and add the paste. Bring up the heat, not allowing it to boil, and whisk until the hot chocolate has thickened a little and is heated through.

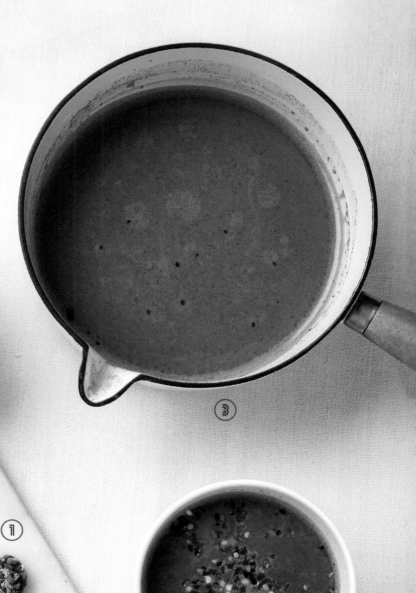

LOLLIES

The first three lollies are fresh juice lollies, packed with vitamins. They make a refreshing and light, sweet end to a meal. I've broken my 'always add protein' rule here, as the quantity that you are having is miniscule and nothing to lose sleep over. Add a handful of nuts if you want to turn any of these into a snack. Do play around with different combinations, adding herbs such as mint and basil. You may find them sweet enough without the stevia, so simply adjust to your taste. Avoid shop-bought concentrate and use freshly squeezed juice. The next three lollies contain protein – from yogurt or milk – again, experiment and play around. I use full-fat Greek yogurt here as 0% tends to form little ice crystals, rather than the creamier texture we're after. These all take 6–8 hours to freeze.

① Lemon & Lime Ⓥⓖ

The devil in you can add a few chilli flakes.

Makes 8

juice of 3 lemons

juice of 3 limes

3–5 mint leaves, to taste (optional)

stevia, to taste

I roll the citrus fruits under the ball of my hand for a few seconds to help release the maximum juice, then squeeze them into a bowl, removing any seeds.

Pop a bit of the juice into a pestle and mortar with the mint leaves and squelch. (If you prefer a less minty flavour, you can just chop the mint for decoration, or leave it out.) Combine this into the remaining juice and taste. Add water and stevia to taste, remembering that you want the unfrozen mixture to taste quite intense. Pour into moulds and freeze for at least 6 hours.

② Blood Orange & Passion Fruit Ⓥⓖ

Makes 8

juice of 3 passion fruits

juice of 3 blood oranges

juice of 1 lemon

stevia, to taste

Squeeze out the passion fruit pulp and push it through a sieve to remove the seeds.

Combine with the orange and lemon juices; you can blend it for a smoother consistency, but it's not essential.

Add water and stevia to taste, remembering that you want the unfrozen mixture to taste quite intense. Pour into moulds and freeze for at least 6 hours.

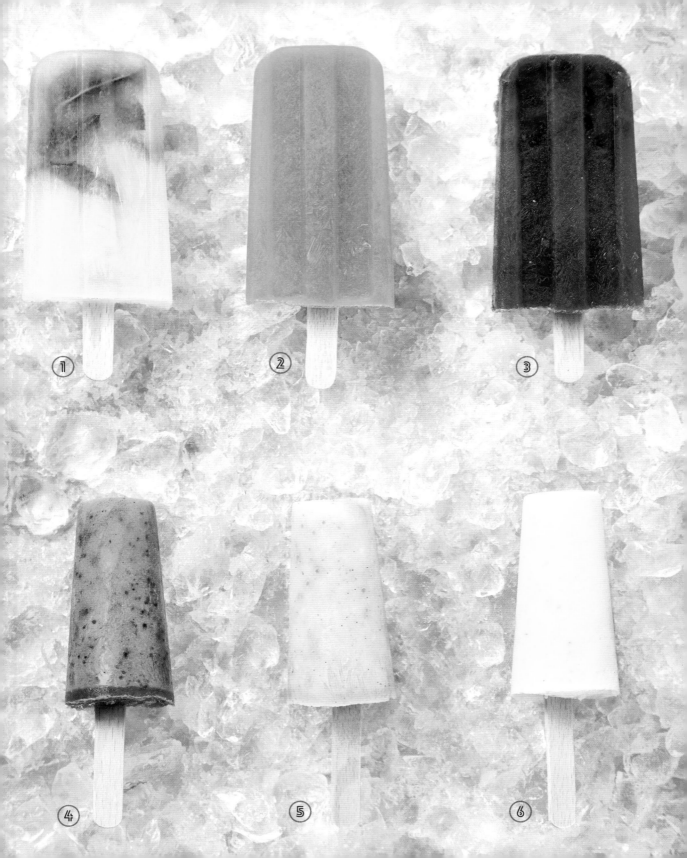

③ Pomegranate & Cherry ⓥg

Makes 8

2 x 200g (about 2 cups) cartons ready-prepared pomegranate seeds

juice of 1 lemon

1 tablespoon cherry concentrate, plus more if needed

200ml (¾ cup) water

stevia, to taste

Combine all the ingredients except the stevia in a high-speed blender and blitz for a minute.

Pour the mixture through a fine sieve and test the flavour. Add stevia to taste or double up on the cherry concentrate for a more intense flavour.

Before pouring into your moulds, sprinkle a few pomegranate seeds into the base for decoration and crunch. Freeze for at least 6 hours.

④ Strawberry & Blueberry Cream ⓥ

Makes 8

250g (9oz) ripe strawberries

100g (½ cup) blueberries

½ teaspoon vanilla paste

stevia, to taste

250g (1 cup) full-fat Greek yogurt

Put the strawberries, blueberries, vanilla and a pinch of stevia into a powerful blender and whizz until you've got a smooth purée.

Now add the Greek yogurt and pulse, just until it is mixed through a little, but still a little marbled. Pour into moulds and freeze for at least 6 hours.

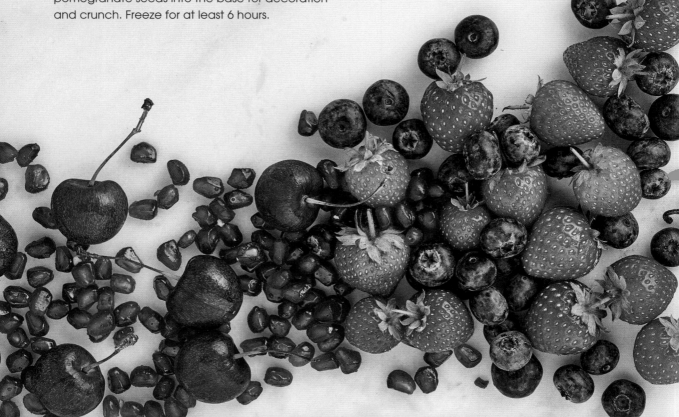

⑤ Vanilla & Banana Mini Milks Ⓥ

Makes 8

500ml (2 cups) full-fat milk

250g (1 cup) full-fat Greek yogurt

½ banana

2 teaspoons vanilla paste

Blend the milk, yogurt and banana until you've got a really smooth purée. Roughly swirl the vanilla paste into the mixture, then pour into moulds to freeze for at least 6 hours.

⑥ Coconut, Pineapple & Lime Ⓥg

Makes 8

400ml (14oz) can reduced-fat coconut milk

juice of 2 limes

1 teaspoon finely grated unwaxed lime zest

200g (about 1 cup) prepared fresh pineapple

stevia, to taste

Blend together the coconut milk, lime juice and half the lime zest until smooth. Add the pineapple and pulse, so that little chunks remain, or blend until really smooth if you prefer.

Taste and add a little stevia if required, but it should be sweet enough. Stir in the remaining lime zest and pour into moulds to freeze for at least 6 hours.

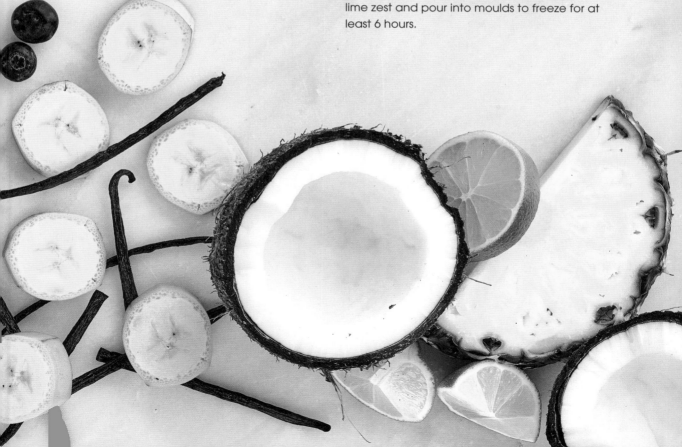

REFRESHING DRINKS

Whenever I've got a glut of citrus fruit, I juice it and either store it in an airtight jar in the fridge, or freeze it in ice-cube trays, so that I've always got a little something on hand to add to water, especially in the evenings when you can miss the ceremony of having a glass of something a bit stronger. Adding lemon and lime juice gives extra zing and strength, so you need less of it. These all keep well as ice cubes and can be added to still or sparkling filtered or mineral water.

① Sweet Rooibos Iced Tea ⓥⓖ

Makes 8 drinks

1 cinnamon stick or 1 cinnamon tea bag

4 Rooibos tea bags

100ml (scant ½ cup) boiling water

1–2 teaspoons stevia, to taste

Steep the cinnamon and tea bags in the boiling water for 1 hour. After steeping, remove the cinnamon and tea bags.

Once cooled, sweeten to taste and freeze in ice-cube trays.

When ready to drink, defrost a cube quickly with a little hot water. Add ice, lemon slices, slices of red grapefruit and mint sprigs and top up with still or sparkling water.

② Lemon & Ginger Sling ⓥⓖ

Makes 8 drinks

2.5cm (1 inch) fresh root ginger, peeled and roughly sliced (adjust to taste)

50ml (scant ¼ cup) boiling water

juice of 8 lemons

1–2 teaspoons stevia, to taste

Steep the ginger in the boiling water for 1 hour, then remove the ginger.

Once cooled, mix with the lemon juice. Sweeten to taste with the stevia and freeze in ice cube trays.

When ready to drink, defrost a cube quickly with some hot water. Add ice and lemon slices. Either top up with still or sparkling water, or serve hot with boiling water.

③ Pink Grapefruit Sours (Vg)

Makes 8 drinks

1–2 teaspoons stevia, to taste

juice of 1 pink grapefruit

juice of 4 limes

Dissolve the stevia in a little hot water. Mix into the remaining ingredients, then store in an airtight jar in the fridge, or freeze in ice-cube trays.

When ready to drink, defrost a cube quickly with hot water and top up with still or sparkling water.

④ Thermogenic Tea (Vg)

Makes 8 drinks

1 cinnamon stick or 1 cinnamon tea bag

1 green tea bag

2 peppermint tea bags

250ml (1 cup) boiling water

1–2 teaspoons stevia, to taste

Steep the cinnamon and tea bags for 1 hour in the boiling water.

Remove the cinnamon and tea bags and sweeten the concentrated tea to taste with the stevia. Freeze in ice-cube trays.

When ready to drink, defrost a cube quickly with hot water. Add plenty of ice, slices of lemon and mint sprigs and top up with still or sparkling water.

⑤ Strawberry Limeade (Vg)

Makes 8 drinks

1–2 teaspoons stevia, to taste

juice of 4 limes

400g (about 2½ cups) puréed strawberries

basil leaves, finely sliced, to taste

Dissolve the stevia in a little hot water. Mix into the remaining ingredients, then store in an airtight jar in the fridge, or freeze in ice-cube trays.

When ready to drink, defrost a cube quickly with hot water, top up with still or sparkling water and serve with extra basil leaves.

⑥ Citrus & Mint Fizz (Vg)

Makes 8 drinks

1–2 teaspoons stevia, to taste

juice of 4 lemons

juice of 4 limes

mint leaves, finely sliced, to taste

Dissolve the stevia in a little hot water. Mix into the remaining ingredients, then store in an airtight jar in the fridge, or freeze in ice-cube trays.

When ready to drink, defrost a cube quickly with hot water, top up with still or sparkling water and serve with extra mint leaves.

⑦ The Perfect Iced Coffee Ⓥ

Makes 1 drink

lots of ice cubes

1 espresso shot

½ teaspoon vanilla paste

semi-skimmed (1 or 2%) milk, or unsweetened soya milk

Fill a large glass with ice cubes to the top. Add an espresso shot – no need to chill – and the vanilla paste. Top up with milk of your choice; I use lactose-free cow's milk, because of its reduced sugar content.

⑧ Orange Cooler Ⓥⓖ

Makes 8 drinks

1–2 teaspoons stevia, to taste

juice of 2 blood oranges

juice of 4 lemons

Dissolve the stevia in a little hot water. Mix into the remaining ingredients, then store in an airtight jar in the fridge, or freeze in ice-cube trays.

When ready to drink, defrost a cube quickly with some hot water. Top up with still or sparkling water and serve with extra orange slices and a mint leaf.

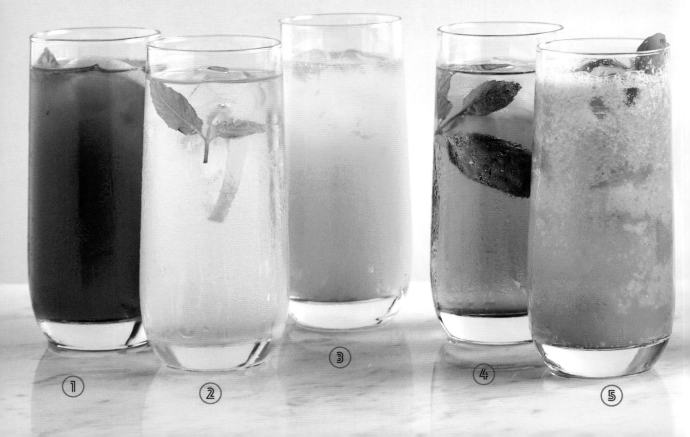

① ② ③ ④ ⑤

⑨ Lemon & Earl Grey Iced Tea ⓥ⒢

Makes 8 drinks

2 English breakfast tea bags

2 Earl Grey tea bags

250ml (1 cup) boiling water

juice of 4 lemons

1–2 teaspoons stevia, to taste

Steep the tea bags for 1 hour in the boiling water. Remove the tea bags.

Mix the concentrated tea with the lemon juice and sweeten to taste with stevia. Freeze in ice cube trays.

When ready to drink, defrost a cube quickly with hot water. Add plenty of ice and top up with still or sparkling water.

⑩ Mujeras Fizz ⓥ⒢

Makes 1 drink

1 lime, quartered, plus a little lime juice

Tajín seasoning (a wonderful Mexican blend of dehydrated lime, chilli and salt, check online for stockists)

a few mint sprigs

Dip the rim of a glass in lime juice in a saucer, then dip into the Tajín seasoning in another saucer.

Using a muddler or long-handled spoon, bash the lime quarters and mint in the bottom of the glass to release the flavours, then top up with ice and sparkling water.

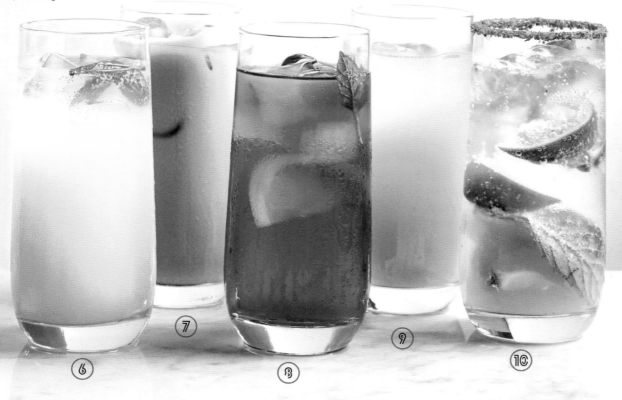

GLOSSARY

UK = US

aubergine = eggplant
baking powder = baking soda
baking tray = baking pan
bavette steak = flank steak
beef tomato = beefsteak tomato
casserole dish = Dutch oven
chickpea flour/gram flour
chicory = endive
chilli flakes = red pepper flakes
clingfilm = plastic wrap
coriander (fresh) = cilantro
coriander (spice) = coriander
cornflour = cornstarch
courgette = zucchini
dessicated coconut = shredded coconut
double cream = heavy cream
fillet steak = tenderloin steaks
greaseproof paper = non-stick parchment paper
ground almonds = almond flour
griddle pan = ridged grill pan
grill = broiler
groundnut oil = peanut oil
king prawn or tiger prawn = jumbo shrimp
kitchen paper = paper towels
minced lamb, beef, pork = ground beef, lamb, pork
natural yogurt = plain yogurt
passata = sieved tomatoes
prawn = shrimp
peppers = bell peppers
rapeseed oil = canola oil
rocket = arugula
romano pepper = long bell pepper
shop-bought = ready-made
single cream = light cream
spring onions = scallions
starter = appetizer
topside of beef = bottom round of beef
vanilla pod = vanilla bean
wholemeal flour = wholewheat flour

Publisher's note

Both imperial and metric measurements have been given in all recipes. Use one set of measurements only and not a mixture of both.

Eggs should be medium unless otherwise stated. The Department of Health advises that eggs should not be consumed raw. This book contains dishes made with raw or lightly cooked eggs. It is prudent for more vulnerable people such as pregnant and nursing mothers, invalids, the elderly, babies and young children to avoid uncooked or lightly cooked dishes made with eggs. Once prepared these dishes should be kept refrigerated and used promptly.

Ovens should be preheated to the specific temperature. All oven temperatures are for a conventional oven. If using a fan-assisted oven, follow manufacturer's instructions for adjusting the time and the temperature. This book includes dishes made with nuts and nut derivatives. It is advisable for customers with known allergic reactions to nuts and nut derivatives and those who may be potentially vulnerable to these allergies, such as pregnant and nursing mothers, invalids, the elderly, babies and children, to avoid dishes made with nuts and nut oils. It is also prudent to check the labels of pre-prepared ingredients for the possible inclusion of nut derivatives.

Vegetarians should look for the 'V' symbol on a cheese to ensure it is made with vegetarian rennet. There are vegetarian forms of Parmesan, feta, Cheddar, Cheshire, Red Leicester, dolcelatte and many goats' cheeses, among others.

INDEX

THE LOUISE PARKER COMPANY

Stroll down Walton Street in the heart of Knightsbridge, and you might well notice a small, but perfectly formed, orange door. Knock three times (or press the buzzer), and you'll find yourself in our first clinic, home to me and my team of dieticians and personal trainers.

For twenty years now, I've been developing and refining weight loss, fitness and wellness programmes for clients who are frustrated with the constant yo-yo of faddish diets and fed up of health gurus scaring them into eating nothing but organic pulses. It is the accumulation of my own personal experience, data and scientific expertise that provides the foundation of The Louise Parker Method.

I'm exceptionally proud of my team, our Method, and the way it can change people's lives, for good. Every day, we coach clients from all walks of life and all over the world, to permanently transform their lifestyles and bodies by following the simple principles outlined in our Method. No fads, no bluff, no madness. Just sensible, tailored programmes designed to eradicate the underlying behaviours that prevent you from leading the life and having the body you desire and deserve.

I don't have a magic wand. The inconvenient truth is that changing your life, your health and your body takes commitment and a little hard work until you get the habit. The good news though, is that our Method is coached by smart, kind empathetic experts who will guide you through the programme, and tailor the Louise Parker Method to you and your lifestyle.

Our Method underpins all our TRANSFORM programmes and continual expert support ensures rapid fat-loss whilst ensuring your metabolism is protected, as well as long-term behaviour change with habits that last forever.

The TRANSFORM programme is available in two formats. Choose 1:1 coaching with your dietitian for 12-weeks of highly personalised, expert support. Alternatively draw on the support of like-minded clients who share your passion to change in our GROUP programme delivered through live weekly webinars.

Whichever route is right for you, our focus remains the same. Expert advice delivered in the kindest, most accessible way to help you permanently recalibrate habits, change your mindset and drop body fat. Coaching is always delivered by registered dietitians and about 40 per cent of our clients are based overseas.

Call us, email or come in to say hello. We'll ask you a few questions and then explain exactly how we can work together to change you, your life, and help you to feel good again.

Louise Parker
81–83 Walton Street
London
SW3 2HP
UK
+44 203 862 5401
info@louiseparker.com

www.louiseparker.com
@louiseparkermethod

ACKNOWLEDGEMENTS

This book has been an mammoth team effort (with no ghost writer) and it is without question that I would not have got it in – just in the nick of time – without the support, love and constant motivation from my bloody incredible family, friends and work family.

I have to say that without Paul, my devoted husband, this book would never have seen the light of day. There were days where I found the juggle of family life, work and writing just so hard – I could not have done it without you. It takes an extraordinary man to pace and steer me and yet not hold back my constant desire to do more. It is such a testament to our marriage that we work, live, parent (somewhat shoddily at times) and still belly laugh each day. I never thought that someone like you would love someone like me. Thank you for loving your four girls with such abandon.

My uniquely brilliant daughters, Sophie, Milly and Chloe. There are no words. Your glorious personalities, empathy and unwavering pride have eased the struggle that I know every mother feels when we've a lot on our plate. 'Keep going Mummy, you can do it' has remained in my spirit throughout. You are my greatest motivation, joy and sense of pride. You delight me every day.

My parents have shown me nothing but support and faith, while inspiring me to strive hard. My late mother glued our international family together with food and love. Daddy, you are the love of my life, you miserable sod. I look up to you like no one else. Thank you for providing me with the greatest foundation for a happy life.

My older brothers Johnny and Rees are ever-present, despite the miles that separate us. I know I can depend on you night and day and I couldn't be without you. It's been a hard year for all of us – I know brighter days are ahead. I don't pick up the phone enough, but know I love you. Thank you for providing me with sisters at long last, the extraordinary Em and Mouse. And most of all my nieces and nephews – each and every one has such a special place in my heart.

How blessed I am to have in-laws I actually crave company with. Nonna, Pa, Nick and Angie – I adore you. I'm indebted to you for your support and your love and babysitting has sustained us through the toughest weekends. You're all bloody marvelous. I know how lucky we are when we sit around the table, laughing our heads off.

My father always said you'd count your best friends on one hand. I'm perhaps still learning and use both. You know who you are. You are my right hand and my left hand and I thank you all for loving me, flaws and all. You are ten incredible humans. (Seven women, two straight men – at time of print – and one very gay man.)

A huge chin chin to Steph, Normski and the boys for consoling me through the most tedious month of writer's block in Portugal, with cold rosé and constant laughter.

I'm blessed to be supported and mentored by so many inspirational people – each of you teaching me a life lesson every time we speak, whether I've asked for it or not. Some are above but I particularly thank Nicky Kinnaird MBE, Dr Dambisa Moyo, Sandi Toksvig OBE, Leslie Zabala, Baroness Anne Jenkin, David Haines, Paddy Padmanathan, Dr Emma Thompson, Gavanndra Hodge, Lady Sarah Stacey, Henadi Al Saleh and last but not least the phenomenal Lindsay Nicholson. You assure me that anything is possible if you just keep getting up.

I thank my agent – the best in the business – Heather Holden-Brown for actually making my books happen. I respect and love you Matron. You are a superwoman. Whoop Whoop to my publishers at Octopus! How you put up with me, I do not know. My empathetic editor, Eleanor Maxfield is the woman that twisted the arms up above to back our Method, and I will always be so grateful to you. All of you are a delight to work with – Kevin Hawkins,

Yasia Williams, Pauline Bache, Caroline Alberti, Karen Baker and Denise Bates.

Huge gratitude to the talented and oh-so-beautiful food stylist Natalie Thomson for your incredible culinary artistry and boundless positivity. Thank you to Linda Berlin for her wonderful styling. God thank Louise Hagger for her amazing food photography – how lucky little me is to work with such experts and I know how hard it was to shoot casseroles in the heat-waves of August.

Thank you to the one and only Chris Terry – possibly one of the finest men I know that just so happens to take a decent picture of me. You're very cool and a fine photographer.

'Behind The Orange Door' on Walton Street live the best work family I could ask for. I'm running out of room to gush but God, thank you all for making us what we are today. I hope you are as proud of the work that you do as I am of you.

Most importantly, I thank each and every client of Louise Parker that has supported us over all these years, spread the word and not been afraid to tell us where we can improve. I owe it all to you. The little things you say to us, the notes, the unexpected calls years later, are what keep us going.

An Hachette UK Company
www.hachette.co.uk

First published in Great Britain in 2016 by
Mitchell Beazley, a division of
Octopus Publishing Group Ltd,
Carmelite House
50 Victoria Embankment,
London EC4Y 0DZ
www.octopusbooks.co.uk

This edition published in 2020

Design & layout copyright © Octopus Publishing
Group Ltd 2016

Distributed in the US by Hachette Book Group
1290 Avenue of the Americas, 4th and 5th Floors,
New York, NY 10020

Distributed in Canada by Canadian Manda Group
664 Annette Street, Toronto, Ontario, Canada M6S 2C8

ISBN 978-1-78472-625-6

A CIP catalogue record for this book is available from the
British Library.

Printed and bound in Italy

10 9 8 7 6 5 4 3 2 1

Publisher's Acknowledgements

Editorial Director Eleanor Maxfield
Art Director Yasia Williams-Leedham
Designers Yasia Williams-Leedham and Geoff Fennell
Senior Editor Pauline Bache
Copy Editor Lucy Bannell
Photographers Louise Hagger and Chris Terry
Illustrator Ella McLean
Food Stylist Natalie Thomson
Food Stylist (for lifestyle shoots) Iain Graham
Prop Stylist Linda Berlin
Hair & Make–up Victoria Barnes
Production Manager Caroline Alberti